MOVING THE WOUNDED

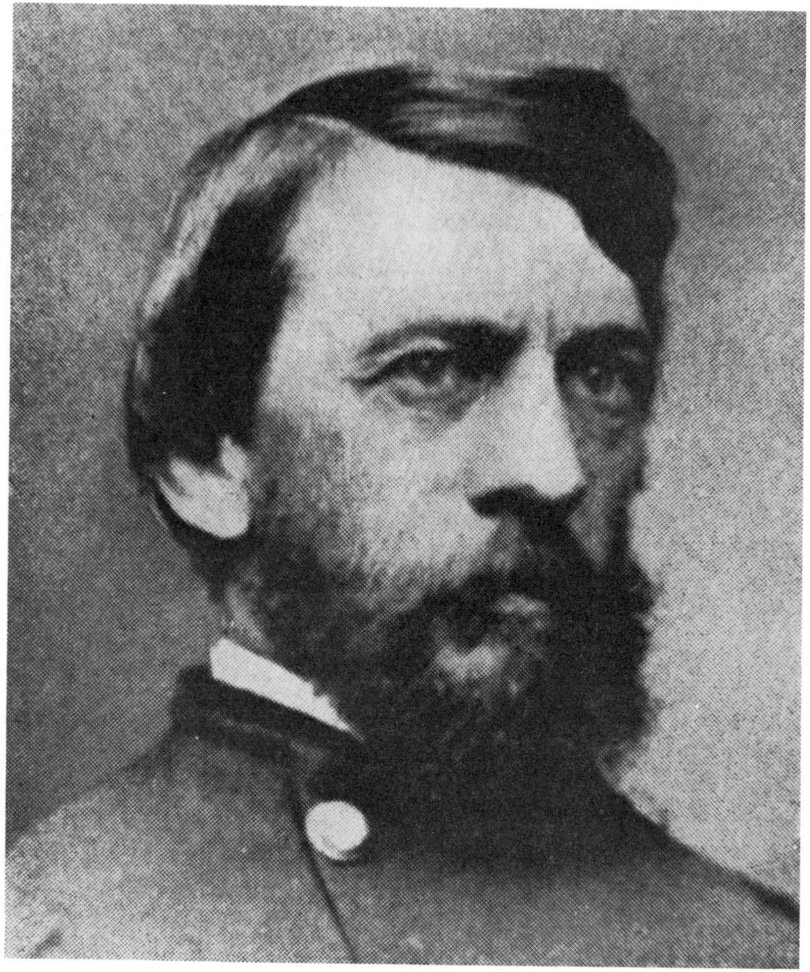

Surgeon Jonathan Letterman, 1824-1872
Courtesy Armed Forces Institute of Pathology, Washington, D.C.

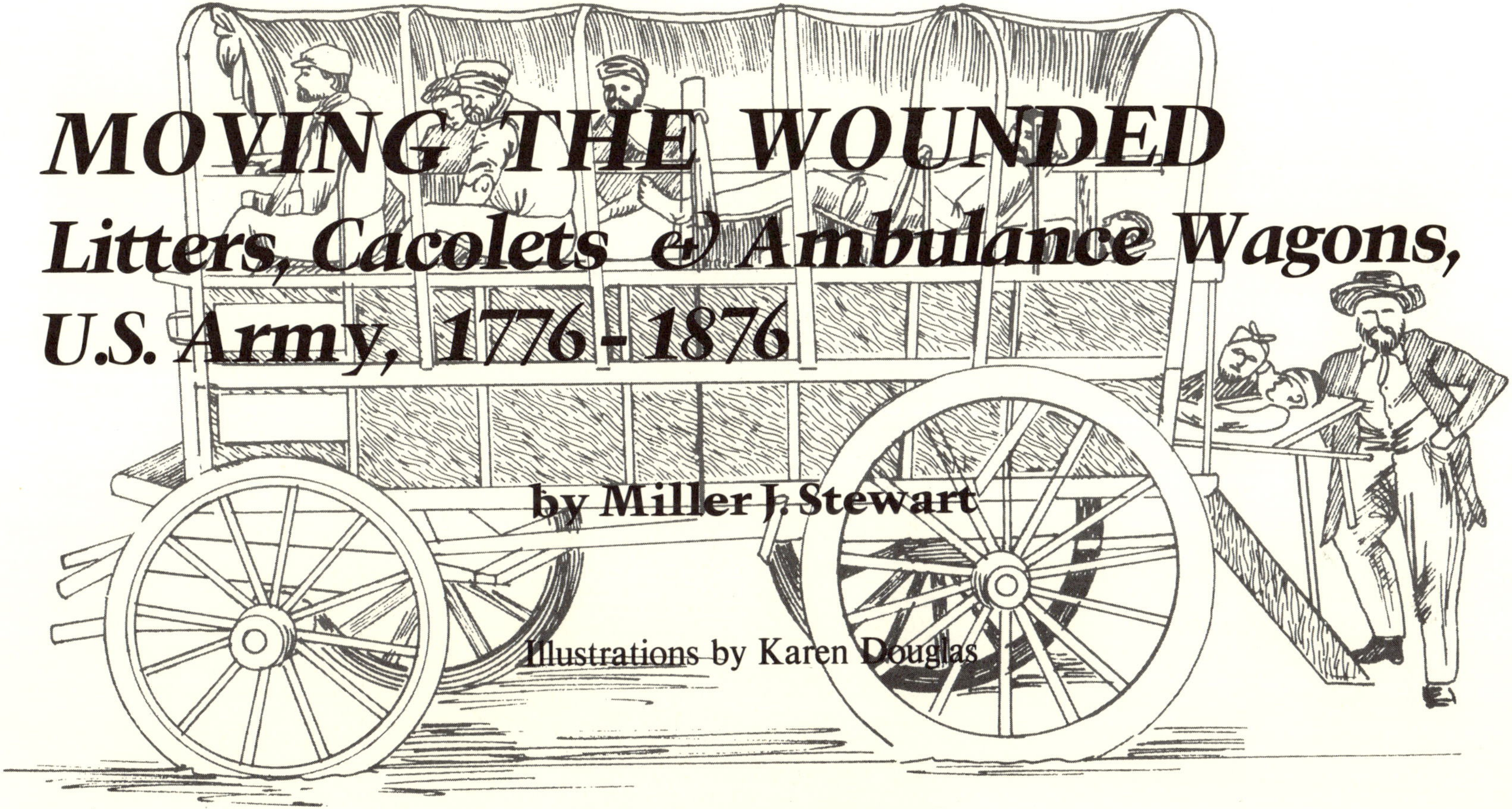

MOVING THE WOUNDED

Litters, Cacolets & Ambulance Wagons, U.S. Army, 1776-1876

by Miller J. Stewart

Illustrations by Karen Douglas

OLD ARMY PRESS

Library of Congress Catalog Card No. 79-83949
ISBN: 0-88342-245-X

Book Design by Leslie A. Johnston

Material cited within the book used with permission of the following:
Larry: Suregon to Napoleon's Imperial Guard by Robert Richardson, John Murray Publishers Ltd. 1974
Doctors in Blue, by George W. Adams, MacMillan and Co. 1952
Civil War Medicine, by Stewart Brooks, Charles C. Thomas, Publisher. 1966
The Medical Department of the U.S. Army in the Civil War, by Louis C. Duncan, a collection of articles from *Military Surgeon*, courtesy of *Military Medicine*, Chevy Chase, MD.
Larrey's *Memoires de Chirurgie de Militaire et Campagnes* (1812), Royal Society of Medicine, London.
Forty Miles a Day on Beans and Hay, by Don Rickey, Jr., University of Oklahoma Press, 1963.

THE OLD ARMY PRESS
P.O. Box 2243
Ft. Collins, CO 80522

CONTENTS

This short history is dedicated to the seldom-known, seldom-credited military surgeons, hospital stewards, litter bearers and ambulance drivers who so heroically labored to alleviate the sufferings of their fallen comrades and, in the words of Baron Percy, "bring them back so that they could become men when they could no longer be soldiers."

ACKNOWLEDGMENTS

No historical research could be undertaken without the untiring efforts of knowledgeable library and archive staffs. In this light, the author wishes to acknowledge the courteous, understanding and valuable assistance of Dr. Elaine Everley and her staff of the Old Army Branch, National Archives and Research Service. The Arizona State University and its Inter-library Loan staff headed by Jane Henning and her assistants, Jewel Hayden and Bobbie Gentry, were most helpful and patient in obtaining hard-to-get research materials. The excellent art work of Karen Douglas is greatly appreciated and acknowledged.

The often tedious, but essential labor of the typists is gratefully acknowledged. Their toil and loyalty transformed the handwritten drafts into the printed word.

INTRODUCTION

Throughout much of history the care of wounded soldiers on the battlefield has been neglected or done so poorly that civilian voluntary associations were formed to perform the task and later to assist the medical departments of the conflicting forces. Even after the development of suitable troop organizations and methods for the removal of wounded from the field of combat the means of transportation might be so traumatic that the patient died of shock enroute to medical care. It was well into the 20th century, with the development of better splints and the application of methods of applying immobilization and traction in the field before moving the casualty, that the mortality began to be lowered. With the advent of motorized transportation the evacuation of casualties became more rapid, but it could still be a rough and traumatic ride from the battlefield over primitive or damaged roads. Only in recent years with the advent of helicopter evacuation has the movement of the wounded soldier from the forward areas become both speedy and relatively non-traumatic.

In the United States, from the times of the Revolutionary War, the types and numbers of wounded in warfare were varied. In guerrilla type actions of the Civil War and in most of the fighting in the Indian Wars only small numbers of wounded resulted from any one confrontation; the troops frequently incurred these wounds far from their home base. In more conventional warfare with large numbers of troops engaged in head-on conflict there were large numbers of wounded, in the thousands, to be collected and given treatment.

For the first type of action with just a few casualties, time permitting, the wounded were given individualized care and were prepared for long journeys back to their home base accompanying their own command. This sometimes required travel over distances of hundreds of miles and taking days and weeks enroute. For the individual wounded in such a situation the means of transport could be most primitive and it sometimes was improvised on the spot. It was not unusual for troops on the frontier to borrow methods proven by the Indians such as the travois. In sparsely wooded country, some expeditions carried long poles to be used for making travois or horse litters; more frequently these were cut in the field as needed. If a friendly settlement was near the patient might be left in a home to be cared for. Sometimes if the command were outbound on a critical mission a small detachment might be left with the wounded, to be picked up on return. On occasions if the importance of the mission justified it or if the safety of the entire command might be jeapordized by delay the patients could be abandoned; rarely the patient was heavily sedated to allow him to die in peace, or a weapon was left with him so that he might kill himself if capture by the Indians seemed imminent.

To properly care for a large number of casualties following a pitched battle between large armies an organized, disciplined and well-trained medical service was needed to quickly collect the wounded, to give life-saving first aid, and then to move the patients to a nearby field hospital where more definitive care could be given by trained physicians and the patient stabilized for further movement to general hospitals remote from the battle area. It was found that an adequate medical service must include a sufficient number of litter bearers readily available and under command of medical department officers as well as plenty of ambulances organic to the medical units. While this had been the general plan in the U.S. Army nearly from its beginning, for years there was no practical organization backed by effective regulations for the medical evacuation of large numbers of casualties. It was not until after the early debacles of the Civil War that an effective medical evacuation system was developed. Even then the capabilities of the Medical Department could be overtaxed following large battles such as at Gettysburg where tens-of-thousands of casualties on both sides lay in the fields for days before they could be collected and put under treatment.

By the end of the Civil War there were adequate supplies and well-trained medical troops to handle the situation, but by the time of the Spanish-American War after years of relative peace or only small conflicts with the Indians, supplies were inadequate for the needs of warfare and many of the lessons of the previous war had to be relearned. This was true to a lesser degree in World Wars I and II. The methods and equipment developed during the Civil War were little changed well into this century with the exception of the substitution of motorized for horse drawn vehicles. In World War II and thereafter the widespread use of blood and blood substitutes, the development of sophisticated portable medical equipment and the use of air transportation for patient evacuation even from forward areas has done much to relieve the suffering of the wounded soldier and to save many lives previously lost.

Miller Stewart in this book has done an admirable job in assembling the known data on the methods and equipment used in the evacuation of wounded soldiers from the battlefield in the military history of this country. He has pictured much of the equipment used and has constructed an informative, interesting and factual story of the evolution of an effective system of collecting and transporting casualties of combat.

James A. Wier
Major General, USA, Ret.

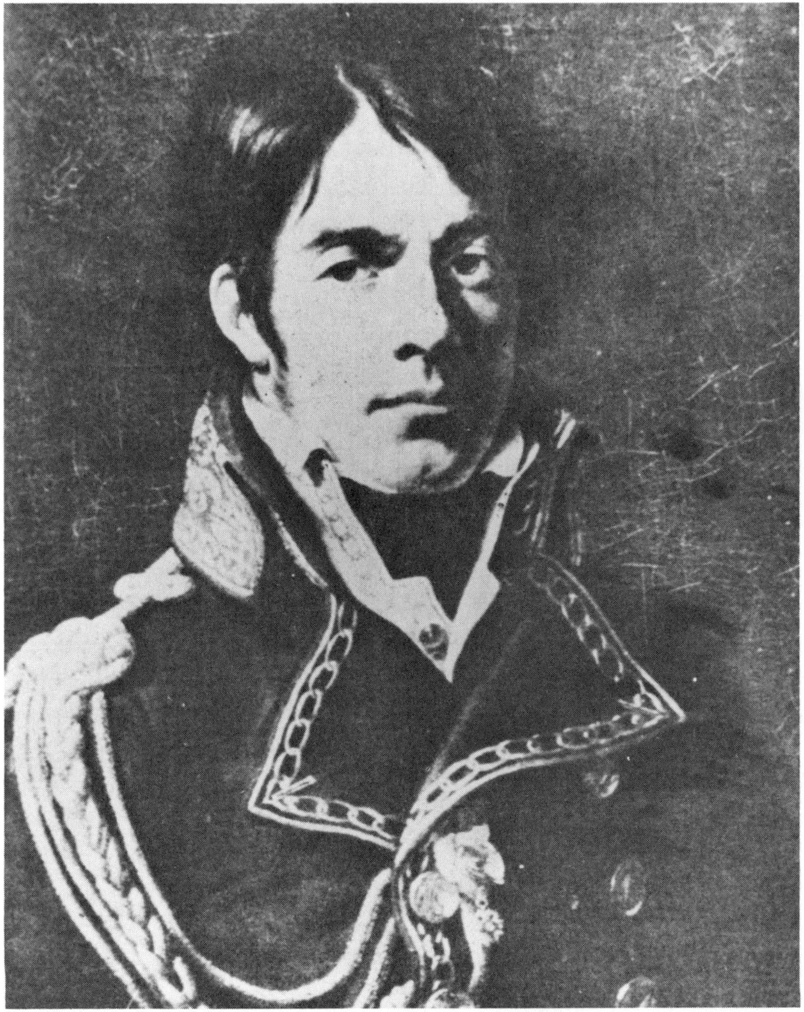

Dominique Jean Larrey
Surgeon to Napoleon's Imperial Guard. (By his friend Anne Louise Gerodet; reproduced by permission International College of Surgeons, Chicago, IL)

Chapter One

EUROPEAN BEGINNINGS

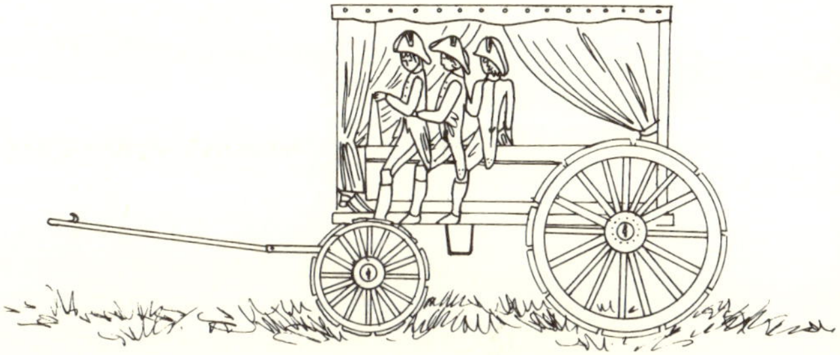

The systematic collection of the wounded from the field of battle only became a reality during the Napoleonic Wars. Far too often, the military commanders, however humane they may have been, were too much concerned with tactics, troop movements and supply to give much thought to their wounded. This gruesome, wearisome chore was left to the military surgeons who suffered frustrating delays because they were not permitted on the battle field until hours after the conflict had ceased. Far too often, the wounded lay for days where they had fallen without water or surgical aid. And added to these melancholy circumstances was the fact that, before the eighteenth century, the surgeons who did accompany the troops were the body servants of the King and the nobility. The rank and file had to look after themselves, or depend upon the kindly arms of their relatives or fellow comrades lest they fall victim to charlatans, rouges and other camp followers.

The first monarch to organize help for the wounded soldiers was Queen Isabella of Spain who in 1487 introduced bedded wagons to carry casualties to large hospital tents set up in safe areas. Her grandson Charles V continued the good work. He stationed doctors among the rear guard with orders to remove casualties to a safe place where their wounds could be safely attended to. But as we have observed, the military commanders only gave perfunctory attention to these orders. They would not digress from their battle plans to consider the plight of their wounded. As a result, the next two hundred years of warfare saw a minimum of help for the shattered soldiers. Casualties were a confounded nuisance and regulations governing their disposal were founded upon that credo.[1]

These regulations required that the ambulances of the time—huge cumbersome vehicles known as fourgons and needing forty horses to draw them in the best of conditions—together with the necessary surgical personnel should wait at least three miles to the rear of any battle action. After the clash of arms ceased these huge clumsy wagons were ordered to proceed at collecting points with all possible speed. Often bogged in mud by their own excessive weight, obstructed by artillery and ammunition trains jammed in all the confusion and disorder of a retreat or advance, these unwieldy wagons never arrived on the scene of battle in less than twenty-four to thirty-six hours after the troops had departed. By that time many who could have been saved were dead or beyond all hope.[2] Truly this was a wasteful use of manpower and demoralizing, too, to the stricken soldier who must wait long agonizing hours for help, as well as to the unwounded fighting men who couldn't be confident of immediate relief.

The situation affecting the wounded had become completely hopeless to the point of utter chaos. Something had to be done quickly—and it was done by two eminent French army surgeons, the Barons Dominque Jean Larrey and Pierre Francois Percy. Their work, as Sir Thomas Longmore pointed out, was so outstanding that their modern plans of removing the wounded from the field of battle by trained attendants in conveyances especially designed for that purpose prevailed in all the continental armies.[3] It is impossible to avoid presenting a short history of the systems they originated and introduced.

Something had to be done—but it needed "a man of exceptional qualities, not the least of which was the strength and will to stand up to the might of military authority." And there was such a man—Jean Larrey.[4]

Dominique Jean Larrey (1766-1842) was a poor shoemaker's son from the small village of Beaudeau nestled in the rugged Pyranees mountains of southern France. The young Jean Larrey came from a family of surgeons who had risen to some prominence in the medical circles of eighteenth century France. It was only natural therefore that the future Surgeon-In-Chief to Napoleon's Armies follow in their footsteps. Jean studied medicine at the Royal Academy of Surgery in Paris, but being nearly penniless was soon forced to accept a post as assistant surgeon in the French navy. From these undistinguished professional beginnings, Dominique Jean Larrey brought a combination of courage, initiative, loyalty, integrity, surgical skills and deep humanity to the task of binding the wounds and saving the lives of Napoleon's soldiers. Larrey awakened mankind's conscience to the inhumanity of war.[5]

Richardson in his biography of Larrey describes him as short, with a slim elegance to his bearing. He wore his thick black hair rather long, in the modern style. His hands were large and strong, reflecting the needs of his chosen profession. His brown eyes mirrored profound intelligence, and practical sympathy for those less fortunate. Truthfullness, utter integrity, pride and stubborness were his guiding principles.[6]

It wasn't until 1792, after experiencing many years of frustrating delays in his attempts to promptly reach the wounded that Larrey was able to introduce his "ambulances volantes" (Flying Field hospitals), capable of moving from place to place like the "flying artillery" of his time. These flying field hospitals included ambulance wagons as we know them.

Here it might be well to observe that the term ambulance is derived from the Latin "ambulare" meaning to move, to march. It is comparable to the old English "marching hospital." Among continental people the term in military phraseology is a hospital establishment moving with the armies in the field and organized to provide surgical assistance to the wounded. In England and America the word is applied to the ambulance wagons and other conveyances by which the wounded are carried to a field hospital or fixed hospitals.[7]

The Flying Ambulance that Larrey designed was a carriage, well sprung and capable of being drawn swiftly by two or four horses. (See Figures 1 and 2.) Under his guidance and with the assistance, both personal and official, of General Jacques Villemanzy, the Army's Quarter-Master General, a few of these conveyances were ready in a short time and put into immediate service. Their first use was in the French advance against the Prussians near Konigsberg. This initial trial of the "Flying Ambulances" was a notable success under the most trying conditions or rough mountainous terrain and heavily falling snow. Here for the first time Larrey was able to dress the wounded in the field of battle before the action broke off and then transport them to safety. Truly a major advance in casualty collection.

Because of the Emperor Napoleon's firm and warm support of his young military surgeon's efforts to perfect the new system of surgical aid to the wounded, his plans for a complete casualty evacuation organization were subsequently brought to a high degree of perfection.[8] It is not necessary to go into the organizational details of these ambulance corps—except to say that each division consisted of approximately 170 men with a chief surgeon in command, (ambulance here, of course, refers to the field hospital and conveyances) and that they were sufficiently staffed to effectively carry out the complete casualty evacuation mission.

A brief description of these carriages shows that the two wheelers (figure 1) resembled the Finley "Two Wheeler" in use in the Union army during the first years of the American Civil War. Larrey's two wheelers resembled old fashioned trunks with the curved tops. Two small windows for ventilation were placed near the top of each side. Double doors at each end facilitated the placing of stretchers in the conveyance. In addition the floor of the carriage could be easily slid in and out for ease in loading patients. This conveyance was roomy enough so that the wounded could be dressed on the floor of the ambu-

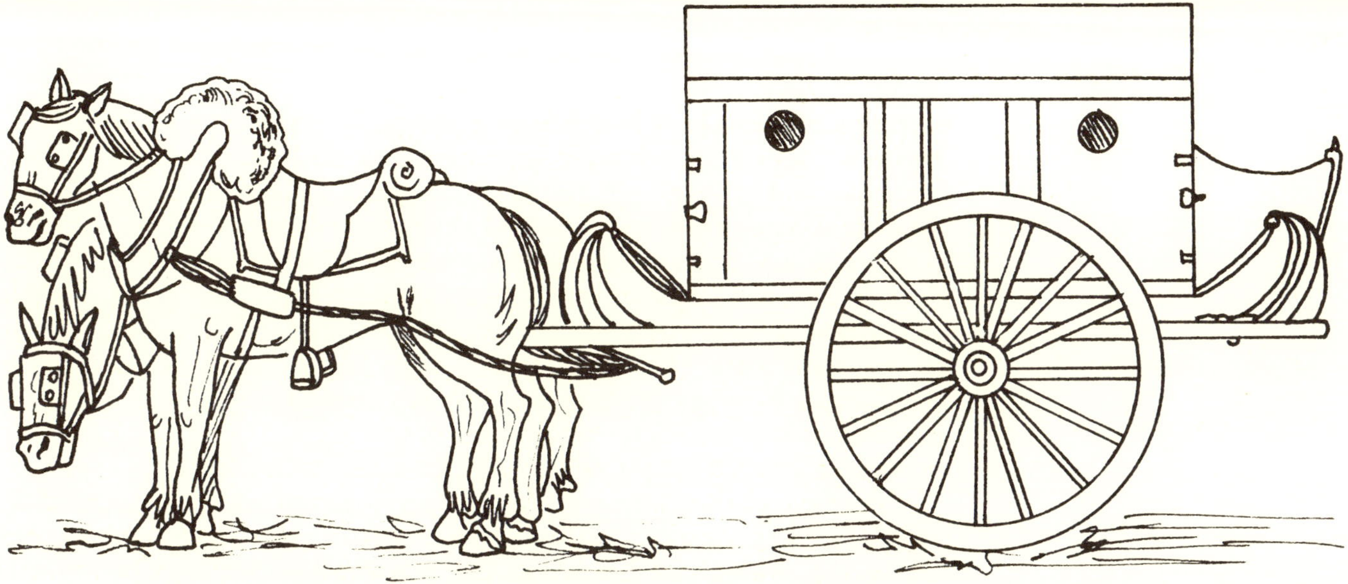

Figure 1-1, Larrey's Two-Wheeled Ambulance

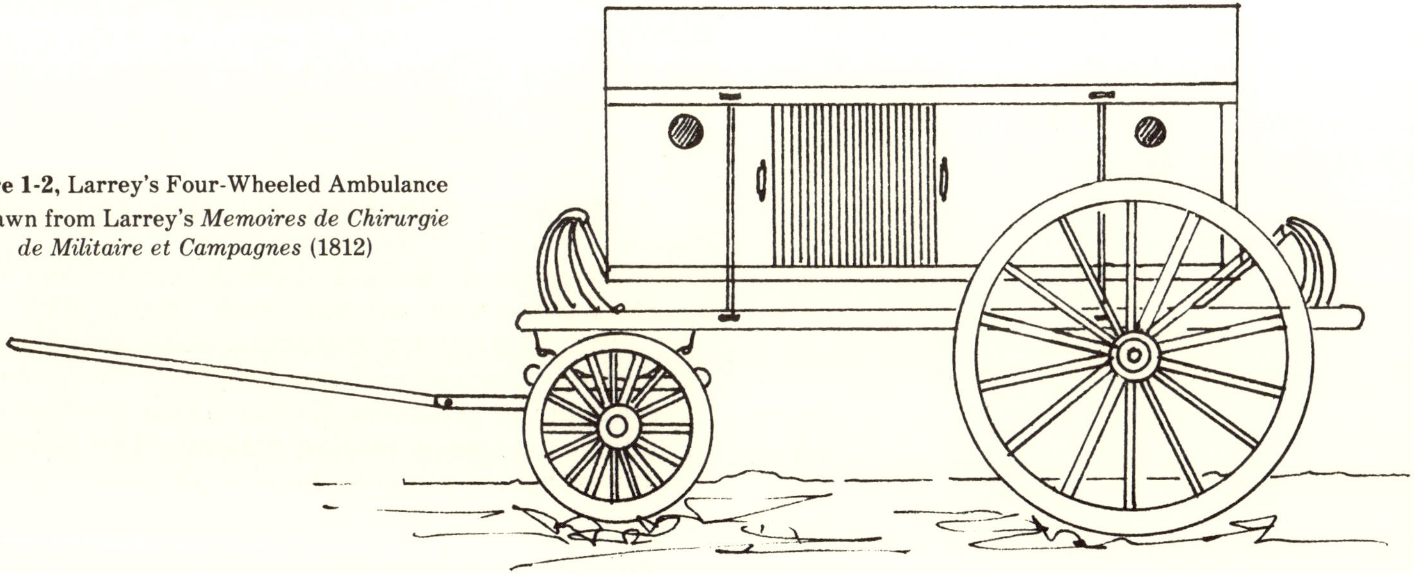

Figure 1-2, Larrey's Four-Wheeled Ambulance
Redrawn from Larrey's *Memoires de Chirurgie de Militaire et Campagnes* (1812)

lance if the weather were bad. The carriage was drawn by two horses—one ridden. By contrast the Union army's "Finley" was drawn by one horse. It was so unsteady that Union soldiers nicknamed it "The Avalanche" because the patients were always liable to be violently propelled from it.

Although essentially similar in design to the "Two Wheeler" just described, Larrey's Four Wheeler (Figure 2) was larger and wider. The floor and mattresses were fixed to the bed of the wagon. Two sliding doors on each side opened to almost full length enabling patients to be easily placed inside. This ambulance could accommodate four reclining patients, however, a bit cramped they might be. Ventilation was provided by two small circular windows on each side. A wheelbarrow slung underneath the running gear served many purposes. This carriage was drawn by four horses, two of them ridden by orderlies. One important feature of this conveyance was its swiveling front axle which permitted ease of maneuverability.[9]

Larrey's colleague and good friend, Baron Pierre Francois Percy, although operating in a different corps of Napoleon's army, was the first to introduce into any army a regularly trained corps of field litter bearers, that is soldiers formed, organized, trained and equipped for the express duty of collecting the wounded while the battle action was going on.

Like Larrey, Baron Percy was an eminent military surgeon who came from a family long serving in the medical profession of France. Percy (1754-1825), while twelve years older than Larrey, was, like him, a courageous and skillful surgeon not afraid to stand up to the military authorities. He, too, worked mightily to bring humanity to the wounded of the wars. Truly, he worked long, hard, diligently and successfully in treating wounded soldiers so that when they could no longer bear arms they could at least be men again.

Figure 1-3, Baron Percy's
Four-Wheeled Ambulance
Redrawn from Larrey's *Memoires de Chirurgie de Militaire et Campagnes* (1812)

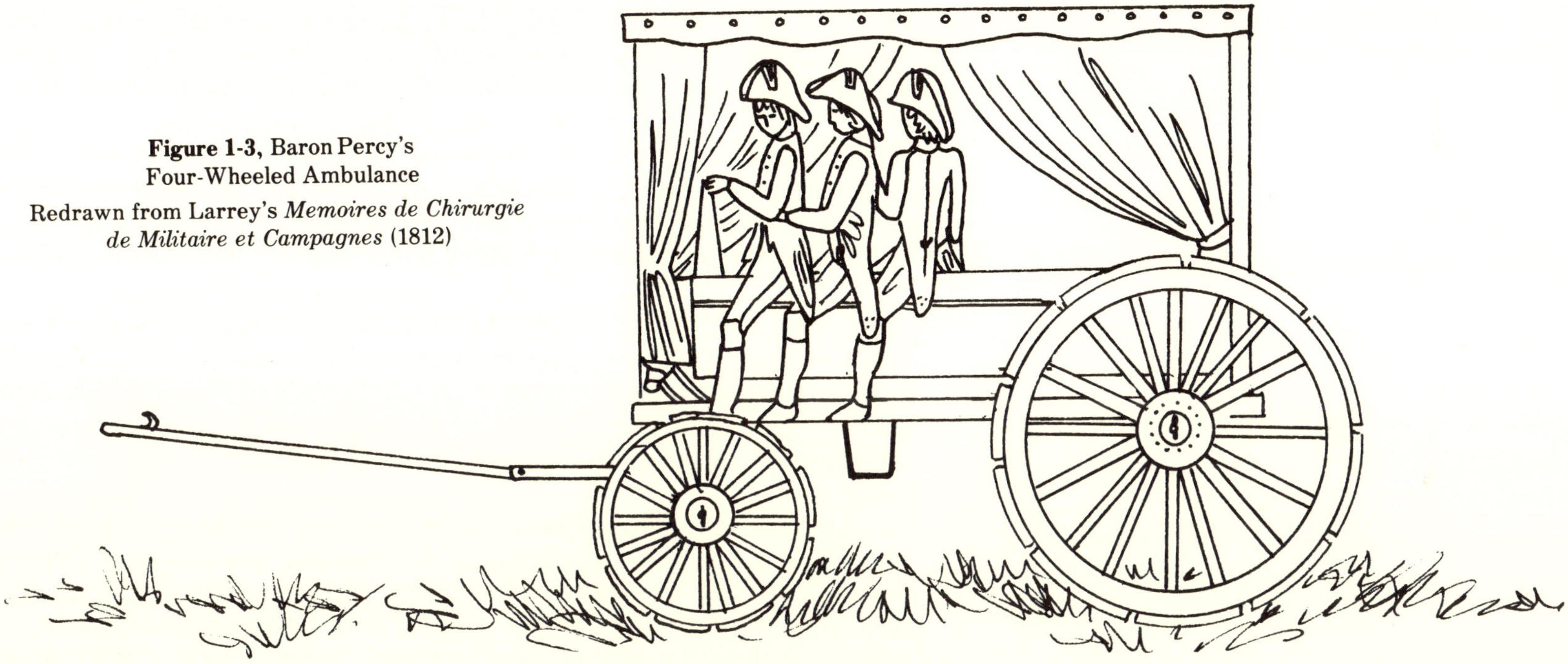

During Larrey's absence in 1799 with Napoleon's forces in Egypt, Baron Percy, then Chief Medical Officer of General Moreau's Army of the North, designed and placed into service a light kind of ambulance capable of rapid movement. It carried all the requirements of a field ambulance in addition to a number of hand litters. (Figure 3)

This conveyance with the peculiar name of "Percy's Wurst," after the German Wurtz, which signified a thick short sausage, or a cylinder, but when joined to "wagen" it signified a long wagon or "wurst wagen." It was quite a startling sight to see the contrivance moving onto the field of battle with eight surgeons sitting one after the other in the main compartment of the ambulance like so many ducks in a shooting gallery. (Figure 3.) This odd appearing conveyance, however, never caught on—it lacked maneuverability, efficiency and could be demolished, wagon, surgeons, equipment and all, by one direct hit from an enemy's shell.[10]

Other continental armies, the Prussians and Austrians, organized, staffed and operated ambulance service to meet their peculiar needs. The Prussians, always well trained, methodical and efficient, formed a specially trained corps of stretcher bearers, something like Percy's. Unlike the French, though, the Prussian litter bearers were equipped with wheeled litters (see Part II). The litter bearers also wore a distinctive uniform and insignia which tended to raise their morale and build esprit de corps in the organization.

It was well into the middle of the 1850's before the British army had any ambulance organization corresponding to that of Larrey and Percy in France. Coupled with the necessity of organizing an ambulance system for its continental armies, the British had to devise ways and means to transport its wounded troops in the many outposts of its far flung empire.

In the Peninsula Campaign of 1808, the British wounded had to be carried from the field by members of the band. This same system of detailing bandsmen as stretcher bearers was adopted, with disasterous results, by the Union armies during the first years of the Civil War.

In fact, both countries, Britain and America, were slow to develop an effective organization for transporting sick and wounded soldiers. The systems in both countries seemingly suffered from the paralyzing effects of tradition-bound military organizations and ineffective medical departments.

From time immemorial, all the best military minds with all the available resources at hand have constantly striven to improve the destructive implements of war and to perfect effective methods to employ them, but until comparatively recent times, only desultory and stumbling efforts had been directed toward the best ways to meet the needs of soldiers disabled by shot and shell. It was as Baron Percy, one of Napoleon's foremost military surgeons, so well explained it, "One would believe that the sick and wounded cease to be men when they can no longer be soldiers."[11]

So as we move westward from the red fields of the continental wars to the forests, mountains and valleys of the American colonies, we find a situation in which large contending armies did not exist; however, the clash of arms between French and British colonists and the protection of hearth and home from the marauding bands of Indians was of great concern. But, these sporadic outbursts did not call for any great concern in the evacuation and care of the wounded.

NOTES

Chapter I

1. Robert G. Richardson, *Larrey, Surgeon to Napoleon's Imperial Guard,* (London: John Murray, 1974) p. 3.
2. Ibid., p. 4.
3. Sir Thomas Longmore, *A Treatise on the Transportation of Sick and Wounded Troops,* (London, Her Majesty's Stationery Office, 1859) p. 25. Sir Thomas Longmore was the authority on the transportation of the sick and wounded of the armies in continental Europe and possibly the world. In addition to serving as a military surgeon in the British Army, Sir Thomas has held the posts of Deputy Inspector General—British Army, Honorary Surgeon to Her Majesty Queen Victoria, and Professor of Military Surgery, Army Medical School, Nettly, England.
4. Richardson, *Larrey,* p. 5.
5. Ibid., p. 7.
6. Ibid., p. 9.
7. Longmore, *Treatise,* p. 8.
8. Larrey was a close and lifelong friend of the Emperor. Upon Larrey's subsequent release from capture at Waterloo, where he was wounded, he became a pensioner of France and legatee of the Emperor Napoleon.
9. Richardson, *Larrey,* p. 37.
10. Ibid., p. 93.
11. Richardson, *Larrey,* p. 2.

Colonial America of the mid-eighteenth century was a geographical collection of separate colonies at peace with the civilized world; dependent upon Great Britain for protection. Militarily, the main threat to their peace was the hostile Indian tribes which were kept in bounds by quickly raised companies of colonial militia.

When the American Colonies did break away from the mother country it was only natural that their army should be organized along the lines of the British military establishment. That being the case, the Continental Army's casualty evacuation system was no further advanced than the British, which still remained shackled to the medieval concept of battlefield casualty removal. In fact, the British Army didn't adopt new means of transporting the sick and wounded until the Crimean War in 1854.

Thus burdened with an antiquated, improvised type of ambulance system, the Continental soldier was not to be afforded the means of quick removal to a place where his wounds could be treated in safety. Hand litters (stretchers), wheelbarrows, ox teams, transport carts, army supply wagons and most anything capable of bearing any weight were used to carry the wounded colonial patriots from the field of strife. If only the military mind of those days could have turned from tactics, logistics, and strategy long enough to consider the plight of their wounded soldiers, the morale of the troops would have been raised and the battlefield deaths lowered.

While the military minds were properly occupied with troop movements, the Medical Department of the Continental Army was showing some concern for the safety of the wounded by issuing directives for the handling of battle casualties. Dr. John Morgan, an early Director General of the Medical department, sent an order to all regimental surgeons stating that they "ought to settle with corps officers what persons are to be employed to carry off the wounded." In addition Dr.

Chapter Two

THE REVOLUTIONARY WAR TO END OF CIVIL WAR

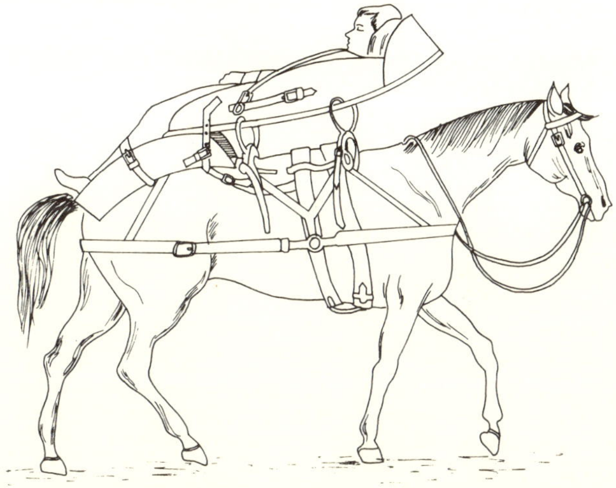

Morgan suggested that regimental surgeons should look to a supply of wheelbarrows or litters to be used in carrying the wounded from the field of battle.[1]

Congress, too, became mildly interested in the plight of the wounded. In one of its early attempts (1777) to reorganize the Medical Department, it gave the Quartermaster General the responsibility to provide a number of "concord waggens [sic], litters and other necessaries for the removal of the sick and wounded." Unhappily, there is no record that such conveyances were ever supplied.[2]

Thus when the agonizing years of the war wound down and approached the fateful fall days of October 1781 at Yorktown, neither the King's men nor the Continental Regulars had ever seen any efficient ambulance service; furthermore neither group would see any until many years later. The British Army would be shackled to the unbreakable chains of the past; the Continental Army would be so reduced in size that a regular organized ambulance service would not be needed because Congress, blind to possible civilized foes, whacked the army down to a mere 700 soldiers, all to be furnished from the various state militias.[3]

Isolated as our military establishment was from the science of warfare in Europe, and coupled with a lack of foreign aggression, one cannot fault the lack of military preparedness on the part of our military planners. Congress, too, might be excused. As a result of this isolation, the new methods employed in the transportation of the sick and wounded which proved so successful in the Napoleonic War were destined to remain on the continent for another generation before the art of warfare in Europe would be given serious study by our War Department.

Thus when a second war against our mother country threatened the peace and harmony of our land, Congress looked to its military cupboard and found it bare. None of the branches of the service were ready for battle action and least of all the Medical Department which had been reduced to six surgeons and seven mates.

Consequently, once again, as in the War of Independence, the wounded had to lay on the field of battle where they fell until some of their comrades came along to remove them to a collecting point by means of crudely improvised hand litters such as those fashioned from army blankets and muskets or the hands of two men clasped so as to form a sort of seat.

It was here at the collecting point away from the field of action that the second phase of casualty removal took place, if enough wheeled vehicles could be found for that purpose. This was of some concern to the military surgeons who oftentimes had to improvise means of transportation so that their patients could get to the hospital as rapidly as possible.

This was amply demonstrated by Surgeon James Mann who, during the War of 1812 near Plattsburg, New. York, transported 450 wounded men on sleighs a distance of some seventy miles losing only six patients by death on the trip to the hospital.[4] Knowing the need for ambulance wagons, Surgeon Mann later requested that the War Department furnish ambulance wagons and teams to the Hospital Corps.

As improbable as it may seem, it was to be in the swamps of Florida during the Seminole War of 1835 that the U.S. Army's wounded were first methodically transported long distances by special ambulance wagons or by two-horse litters. The organizer of this ambulance system was Surgeon Richard S. Satterlee, U.S.A.[5]

In his report to the Surgeon General, Satterlee related that the less severely wounded were carried from the battlefield to the hospitals in supply wagons converted to ambulance service, a distance of some 150 miles "with little inconvenience to the patient." Because of rough roads, however, the seriously wounded were brought out on two-horse litters constructed on the spot. (Figure 2.1.) These two-horse litters proved so comfortable and so well adapted to the rough terrain that Surgeon Satterlee requested the Quartermaster construct twenty such conveyances for future use.[6] However, records do not show that the surgeon's request was ever honored.

To put use of wheeled ambulances in proper perspective, it should be pointed out that wheeled vehicles could not operate under all battle conditions as oftentimes engagements took place in heavily wooded areas, ravines, mountain slopes and other sites inaccessible to wheeled vehicles. In these situations, litters borne by man or animals were the only effective means of transporting the wounded to collecting points.

During the same war in Florida, an inventive minded army officer, Captain H.L. Thistle of the Louisiana Volunteers, devised a single-horse litter for the transportation of wounded men through narrow defiles and over rough terrain (complete description in Chapter IV). Also, it is worthy of note that the ingenious Captain Thistle received favorable mention from the Quartermaster General, Thomas Jesup, for an improvement that he had made on his carbine which apparently corrected a most bothersome defect.[7]

During the next ten years, before the outbreak of the Mexican War, Congress did, reluctantly, increase the military establishment by the addition of a few regiments, but by and large, the aggregate strength of the army remained far below the level it needed to adequately defend the nation against a determined foreign foe or to even keep the peace in the newly acquired territories of the far west.

The experiences in the war with Mexico, 1846-48, did little, if anything, to materially provide for an adequate ambulance service. In fact, ambulance wagons as such were not attached to the American

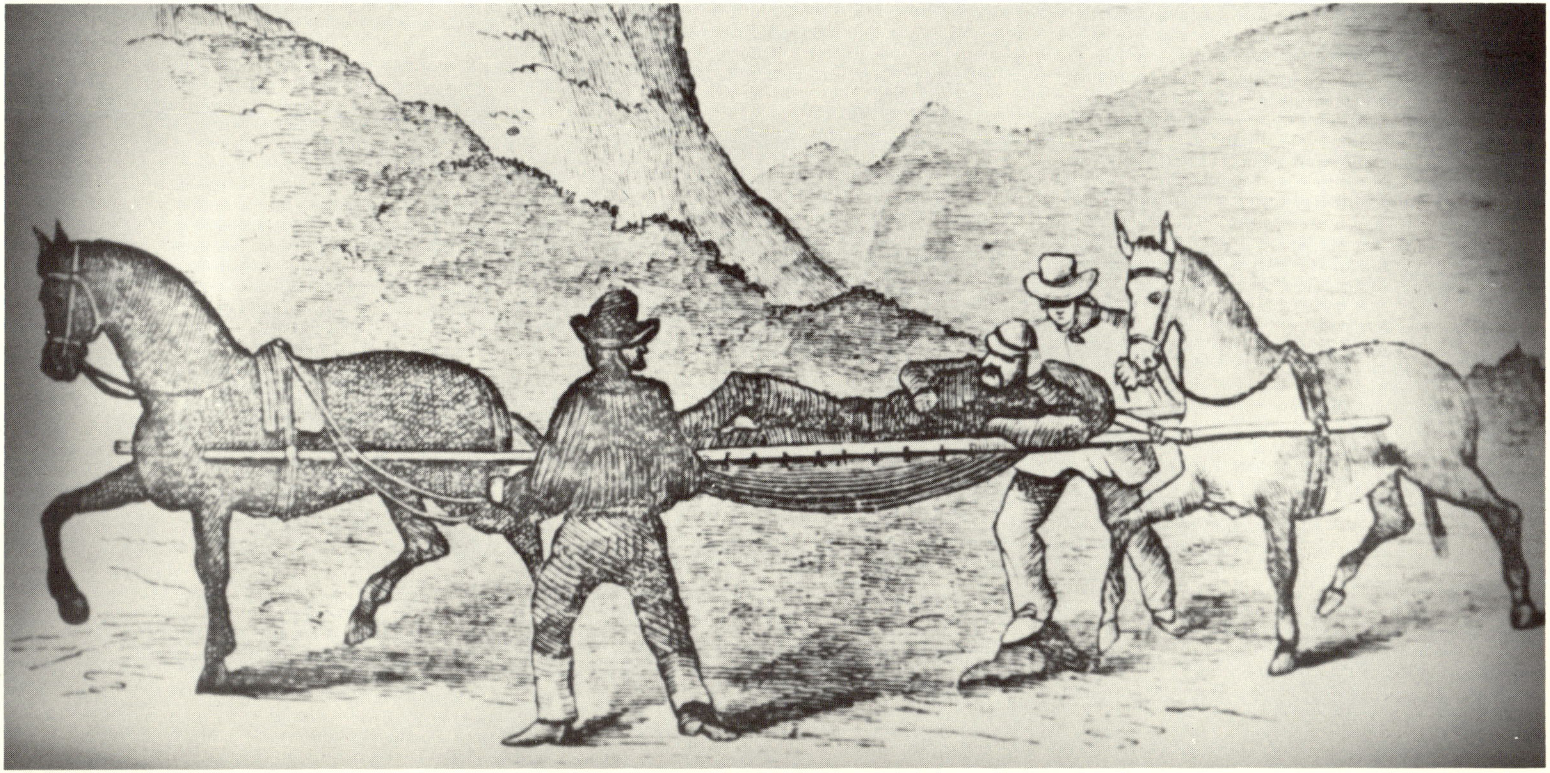

Figure 2-1, Two-Horse Litter

From Marcy, *Prairie Traveller* as depicted in Otis, *Transportation Sick and Wounded Troops by Pack Animals,* S.G.O. Circular No. 9

Army, although Army regulations (1847) did provide that a wagon be attached to the rear guard of a regiment for the accommodation of the sick and wounded, and that when necessary and practicable, the surgeons could render whatever assistance they deemed necessary to "alleviate the pains of the wounded."[8] These regulations, although but one hesitant step forward, recall the ambulance system of Queen Isabella some four centuries before, and it certainly doesn't begin to approach the effectiveness of Larrey's "Flying Ambulances" of Napoleonic War fame.

After the end of the Mexican War, the interest of the army up to 1861 was largely occupied with expeditions and skirmishes against the western Indian tribes, hence, an organized ambulance service was of little concern, as casualties could easily be removed by improvised litters made on the spot. Yet, battle capabilities of the Army engaged the minds and the thinking of a small coterie of officers such as Captain George B. McClellan and Major Richard Delafield led by the Secretary of War, Jefferson Davis. They believed that the Army needed new ideas for it to be an effective fighting force and naturally looked to the European armies for help. Accordingly, in 1854, Mr. Davis appointed a military commission headed by Major Delafield, and including Captain McClellan, to study first-hand the art of warfare in Europe. The observations of this mission to Europe during the Crimean War were published in two reports and covered organization, fortifications, field tactics, weapons, equipment, supply and ambulance trains.

The observations of Major, later General Delafield, Corps of Engineers, in the most approved ambulance conveyances and other appurtenances of the ambulance train provided our military leaders with much useful information upon which to base the transportation of our wounded soldiers in time of war.

According to Major Delafield, the most expeditious means of

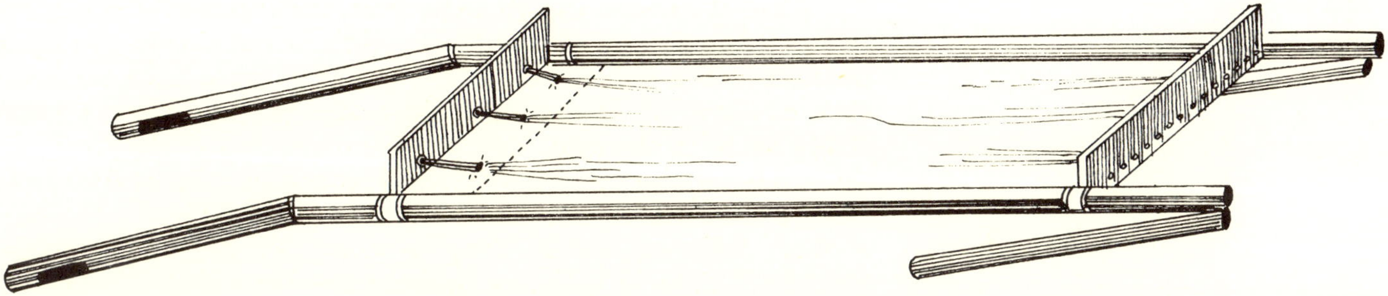

Figure 2-2, Regulation U.S. Army Two-Horse Litter
Redrawn from Otis, S.G.O. Circular No. 9

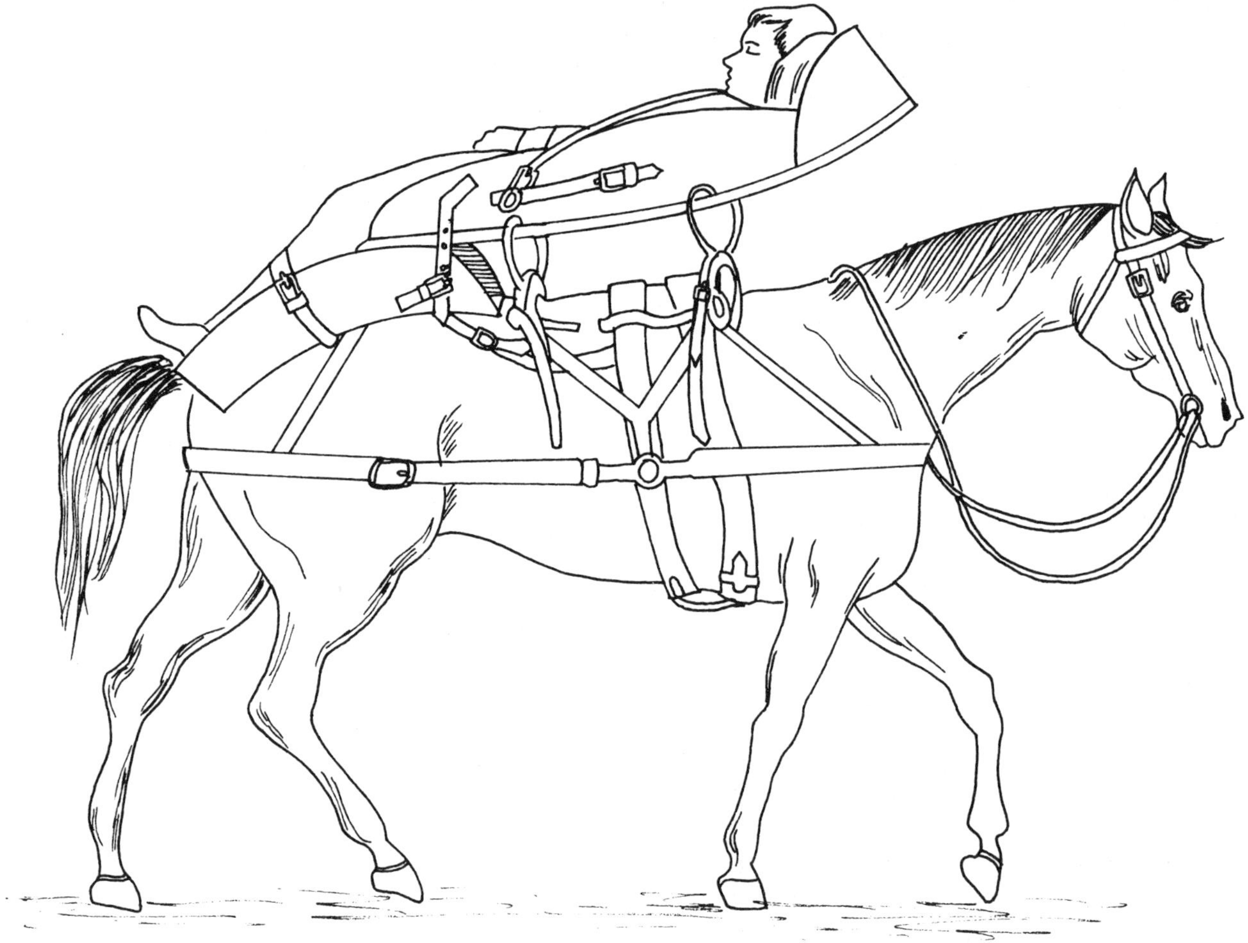

Figure 2-3, Thistles' Single-Horse Litter, 1837
Redrawn from Otis, S.G.O. Circular No. 9

transport with the least number of animals, wagons and attendants combined with the greatest comfort for the wounded soldiers was the number one principle. A second consideration was that the design of the ambulance transports should be such that they can be used on any battlefield whether at the bottom of a valley, on a steep hillside, in a ravine or over ploughed ground, and still transport the seriously wounded with ease and comfort.[9]

Delafields's report together with the practical knowledge of our army surgeons and officers gained in the Indian wars of the west gave much needed impetus and encouragement to our War Department's study of ambulance conveyances. In fact, after Delafield's report became public knowledge the War Department was so besieged by private citizens with their designs of litters that the Secretary of War was moved to convene a board of medical officers to examine and report on the large number of designs submitted.

This board consisting of Army surgeons Clement A. Finley, a sixty-year-old veteran of the Medical Department and later Surgeon General during the first year of the Civil War, Richard S. Satterlee, Charles S. Tripler, later Medical Director of the Army of the Potomac, John M. Cuyler and Assistant Surgeon Richard H. Coolidge, assembled in Washington on November 1, 1859 for the first of some seventeen meetings.

After careful examination, the board disapproved all of the ambulance models that had been submitted. It then issued a statement declaring the importance of completely revamping the Army's ambulance system and requested that the Board be given authority to consider and report upon an ambulance system which it felt would meet all the exigencies of the service. This request being granted, the Board at its seventeenth meeting in late November passed a series of resolutions which were incorporated in the Revised Army Regulations of 1861.[10]

These regulations which remained in force for the duration of the Civil War provided that on marches and in campaigns against Indians, commands of less than five companies were to be allotted one two-wheeled ambulance per company (an infantry company of this period consisted of not more than eighty enlisted men and officers), a battalion of five companies one four-wheeled ambulance, and five two-wheeled ambulances, while regiments were allotted ten two-wheeled ambulances.

The Regulations of 1861 further provided that these allotments would be increased if a state of war "with a civilized enemy" should occur.[11]

It is of interest to observe that paragraph 1296 of the Regulations, which stated that ambulance wagons were to be used *only* for the transportation of the sick and wounded, was honored more in the breach than in the observance. The flagrant disregard of this provision by certain commanders caused a great shortage of sorely needed ambulances as well as adding to the woes of the supply officers who had to see to the repairing of many broken-down vehicles.

Back at the War Department, harassed officials were overwhelmed by the large number of litters and ambulances of various designs ranging from those copied openly from the descriptions in Major Delafield's report to quaint and curious designs of the inventors themselves. Many of these citizens were no doubt activated by motives of patriotism and humanity. Be that as it may, this brief period of concentration on ambulances, litters and cacolets was shattered, when in the early morning hours of April 11, 1861, South Carolina's venerable Edmund Ruffin, arch secessionist, pulled the lanyard on one of the Confederate guns trained on Fort Sumter and irrevocably plunged the nation into four years of deadly destructive warfare.

And as we shall see, an effective ambulance system would emerge from all of the chaos created by the sound of the guns.

NOTES

Chapter II

1. Duncan, Lt. Colonel Louise C. *Medical Men in the Revolution 1775-1783*, p. 121.
2. *The Medical and Surgical History of the War of the Rebellion 1861-1865*, Vol. 2, Part III, p. 944 (hereinafter referred to as OR.).
3. Tobey, James A. *The Medical Department of the Army*, p. 7.
4. OR, p. 944.
5. Otis, General George A. "Transportation of the Sick and Wounded by Pack Animals," Circular No. 9, Surgeon General's Office, p. 3.
6. Otis, p. 4.
7. *Office of the Quartermaster General*, Letters Sent, RG 94, Entry 289 (National Archives and Research Service).
8. OR, p. 944.
9. Delafield, Major Richard. "Report on the Art of War In Europe, 1854-56." U.S. Congress, Sen. Ex. Doc. No. 59, p. 68.
10. Otis, p. 5.
11. Army Regulations, 1861, par. 1294, 95, 98.

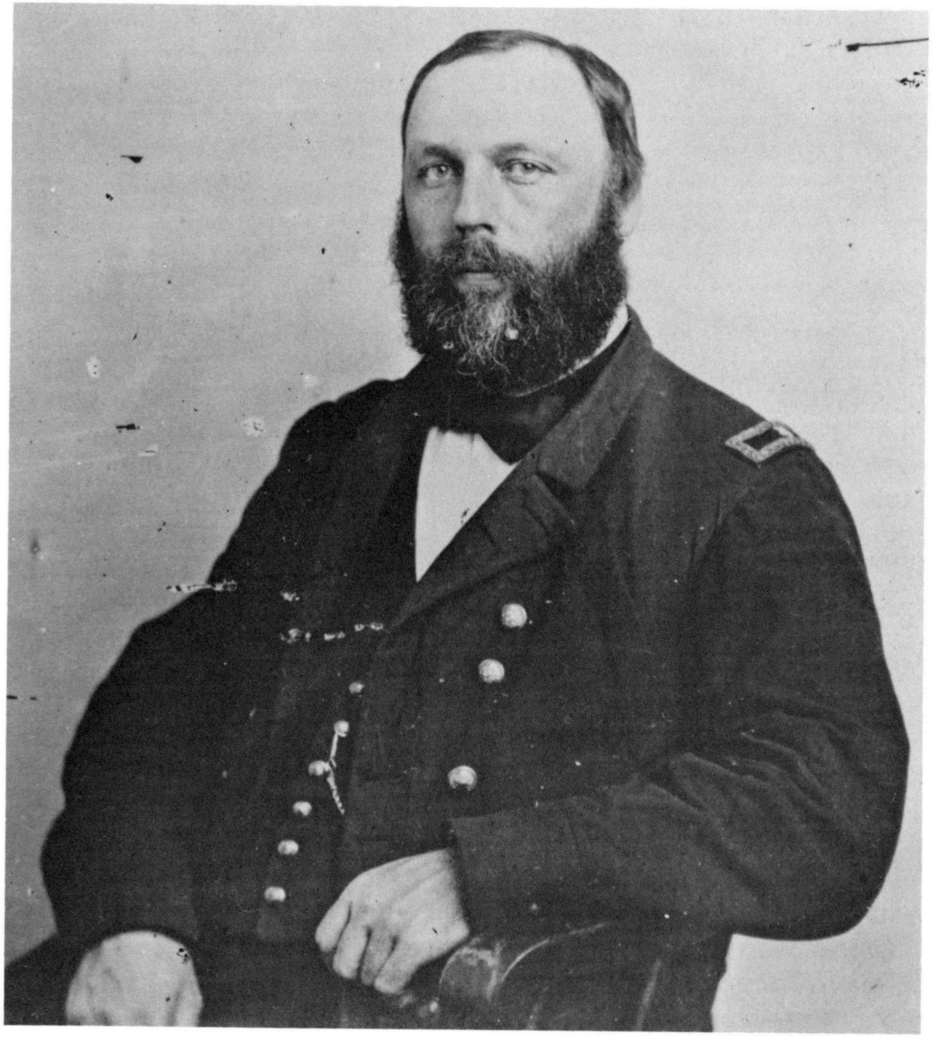

Figure 3-1,
Surgeon William A. Hammond
The Surgeon General, 1862-1864
U.S. Signal Corps Brady Collection, National Archives

Chapter Three

THE GREAT CONFLICT

"Wars Do Exact a Heavy Fee—
But We Do Learn." —*Brooke*

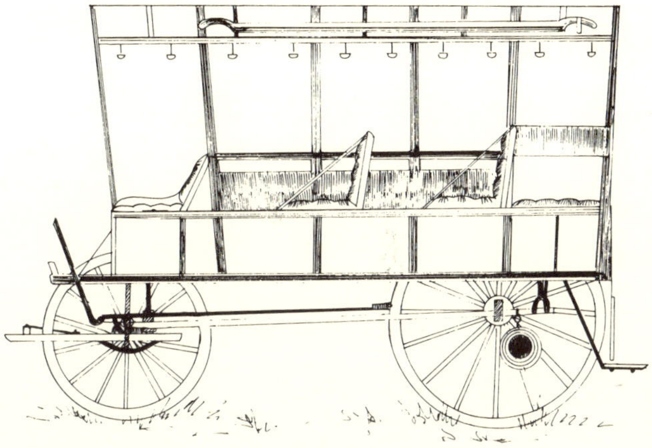

Fort Sumter fell on Sunday, April 14, 1861. Brigadier General Pierre G.T. Beauregard, Commander of the Confederate batteries overlooking Charleston Harbor, had offered the garrison's commander generous terms. The two commanders were old friends; General Beauregard when a cadet at West Point had studied artillery tactics under Major Robert Anderson. The small besieged garrison proudly, sadly, marched out as the band played "Yankee Doodle" and a 50-gun salute added its booming benediction to the occasion. The next day President Lincoln called for 75,000 militia.

And again Congress looked to its military cupboard and found it, as usual, bare. The Regular Army numbered fewer than 16,000 officers and enlisted men, mostly scattered in small commands, policing a territory extending from border to border and coast to coast. And to make matters worse, these commands were poorly trained and poorly supplied. The Medical Department was no exception, in fact it was moribund.[1]

They had neither plans, personnel nor equipment for collecting the wounded or transportation to carry them to hospitals. The resolutions of the Medical Board of Officers, 1859, had not yet been embodied in Army Regulations. In the Surgeon General's Office, seniority promotion, lack of retirement for age or disability, filled the upper ranks with "fossils" who either could not or would not take the aggressive action needed to prepare for an eventual war. When Surgeon General Thomas Lawson, who is purported to have thought it foolish to buy medical text books, died, he was succeeded by Surgeon Clement A. Finley, another relic of the 1812 period. Finley, born a few years before the dawn of the nineteenth century, had entered the Army as a Surgeon's Mate in 1818, so that by the beginning of the Civil War he was overdue for retirement. At the time of his appointment, he was described by one observer as "handsome, complacent, and self satisfied." He was "vain and incompetent" according to Frederick Law Olmstead, prominent member of the prestigious U.S. Sanitary Commission.[2] He had few ideas of his own, but was always quick to squelch others.[3] However, be that as it may, Finley's tenure was short lived; the Sanitary Commission forced his retirement by April 1862.

For his replacement, the Secretary of War passed over many senior officers to select Assistant Surgeon William A. Hammond for the position. Surgeon Hammond, at thirty-four years of age, brought keen intelligence, great common sense, vigor and vison to the formidable tasks that would be needed to put the Medical Department on a war footing.[4]

The years 1861 to late 1862 were years of frustration for the Medical Department. Shortage of ambulances, poorly trained stretcher bearers, and undisciplined drivers continually hampered the Medical Department's mission—proper care for the wounded.

The first, shortage of ambulances, was glaringly evident at the first Battle of Bull Run (July 21, 1861). One regiment (600-700 men) of the First Connecticut Volunteers had only one four-wheeled ambulance, no hand litters, few hospital supplies and a few scared untrained bandsmen to care for the wounded.[5] These unfortunates had to depend upon friends and relatives to pick them up and take them to a nearby farm house or drive them back to Washington. In fact, for months to come and on other battlefields, to a degree, the family carriage became a symbol of both hope and despair. Many soldiers from this first battle were compelled to drag their shell-torn bodies back to Washington some twenty-five miles, because the ambulance service had been so poor.

General George B. McClellan, who took to the field (March, 1861) after months of organizing and disciplining the large Union army, should not have had any medical problems, but bad teamwork and a

Figure 3-2, Two-Wheeled Finley's and Four-Wheeled Tripler's. *U.S. Signal Corps Brady Collection, National Archives*

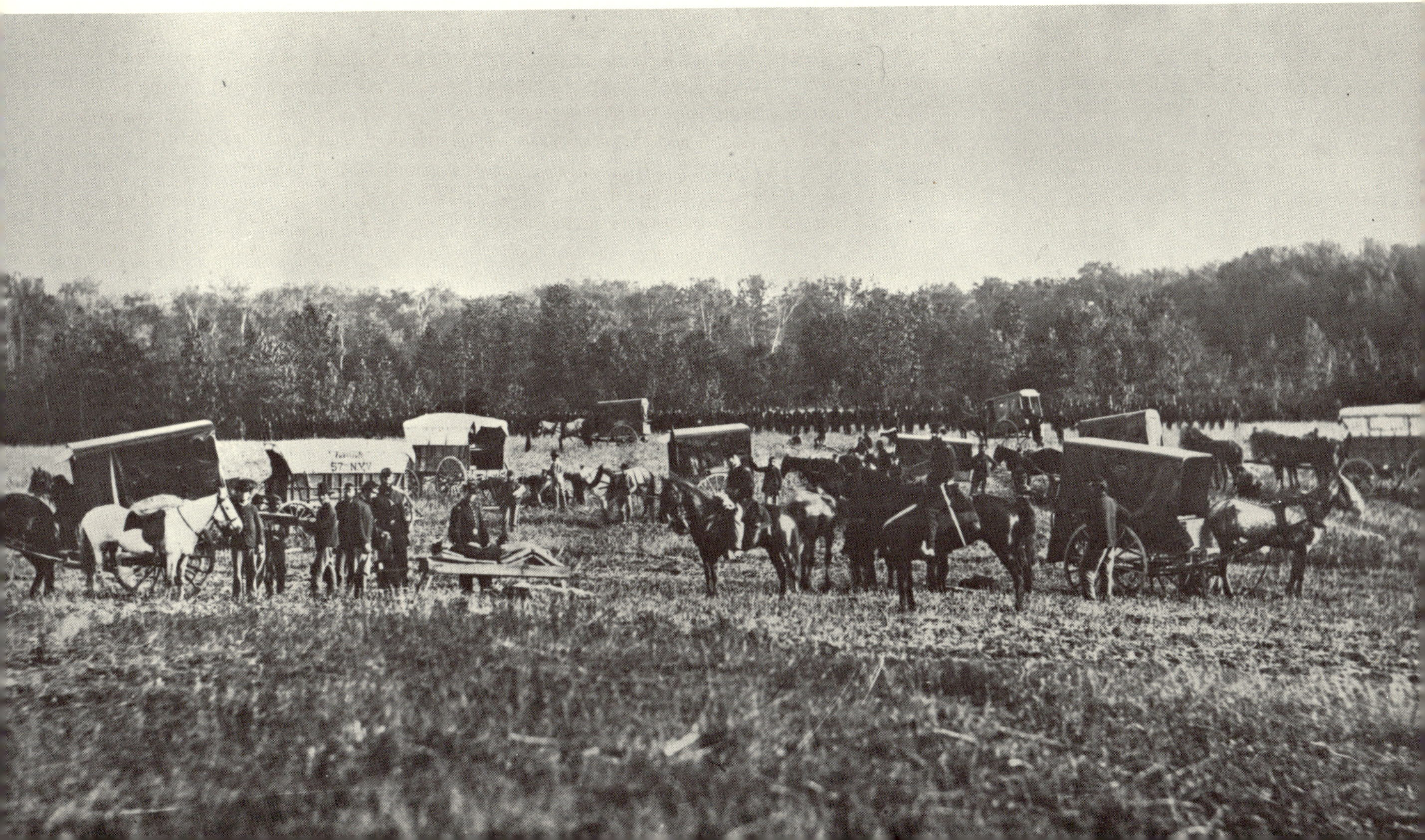

dearth of ambulances made a mess of the medical services. This army left the Washington area with 177 ambulances, seventy-three short of Surgeon Tripler's request. One single ambulance in one of the brigades could not be found to transport a sick colonel to the hospital. This sorry picture of shortages continues. Toward the end of the Peninsular Campaign, an army corps of some 30,000 men had ambulance transportation for a mere 100 men.[6] McDowell's corps, which was supposed to have three ambulances to each regiment, actually counted forty-one for the entire thirty-three regiments, and this corps was said to have been the best supplied.[7]

At the particularly hard fought battle of Wilson's Creek (August 10, 1861), the wounded could not be moved for five or six days because of the acute shortage of ambulances. Surgeon John H. Brinton, Medical Director of General Grant's forces in the west, reported from Belmont, Missouri (November 7, 1861) that he was forced to abandon the wounded because he had no ambulances.[8]

Shortages such as these could easily be multiplied by reviewing reports from other armies, corps, brigades and regiments. Part of the blame for these shortages could be attributed to improper requisitions by newly appointed unit quartermasters, or by slowness in contract and manufacture. Another more immediate cause was that the Quartermaster Department controlled issuance of ambulances and assignment of civilian drivers to the Medical Department.

Among the Confederate forces the ambulance system, patterned from that of the Federal Army, was poor from the start and became hopeless toward the end of the war. For example, during 1863 the inspecting officers reported only thirty-eight ambulances in the whole Confederate Army in Mississippi. By 1865 not one ambulance could be found in an entire brigade in the Department of West Virginia and East Tennessee.[9]

The second obstacle that faced the Medical Department was that of poorly trained stretcher bearers. This vexatious problem showed up at the chaotic Battle of Bull Run. These stretcher bearers, whose duty was the removal of the wounded to collecting stations, were selected from the regimental musicians and convalescents temporarily detailed for that duty. But scrubbing blood-soaked floors and tables, disposing of dirty scabby bandages and carrying bleeding shell shocked soldiers had nothing to do with music, accordingly the impressed musicians fled the scene. Time and time again battlefield commanders charged that these rascally fellows "proved utterly worthless in bringing off the wounded, behaving with utmost cowardice, and it required more persons to watch and see that they did their duty than their service was worth." This complaint was echoed by another regimental commander who angrily reported that they were "averse to labor or danger and habitually insubordinate."[10]

In an effort to correct this distressing problem, Surgeon Charles S. Tripler, Medical Director of the Army of the Potomac, set up an organization of stretcher bearers who were to be under the direct supervision of brigade surgeons and were to be drilled every day, except Sunday, in all phases of handling and caring for the wounded.[11] However, these stretchermen would not be fully efficient nor properly selected until the advent of Surgeon Letterman.

The third obstacle to speedy transportation of the wounded to hospitals was the vast number of civilian lay abouts hired by the Quartermaster Corps to drive the horse-drawn conveyances. Practically every one of these villianous fellows hired for the Second Battle of Bull Run (August 29, 1862) fled the scene of bloodshed. The removal of the wounded became so desperate that Surgeon General Hammond was compelled to commandeer vehicles from the streets of Washington. By heroic efforts he managed to round up 140 hacks, forty busses

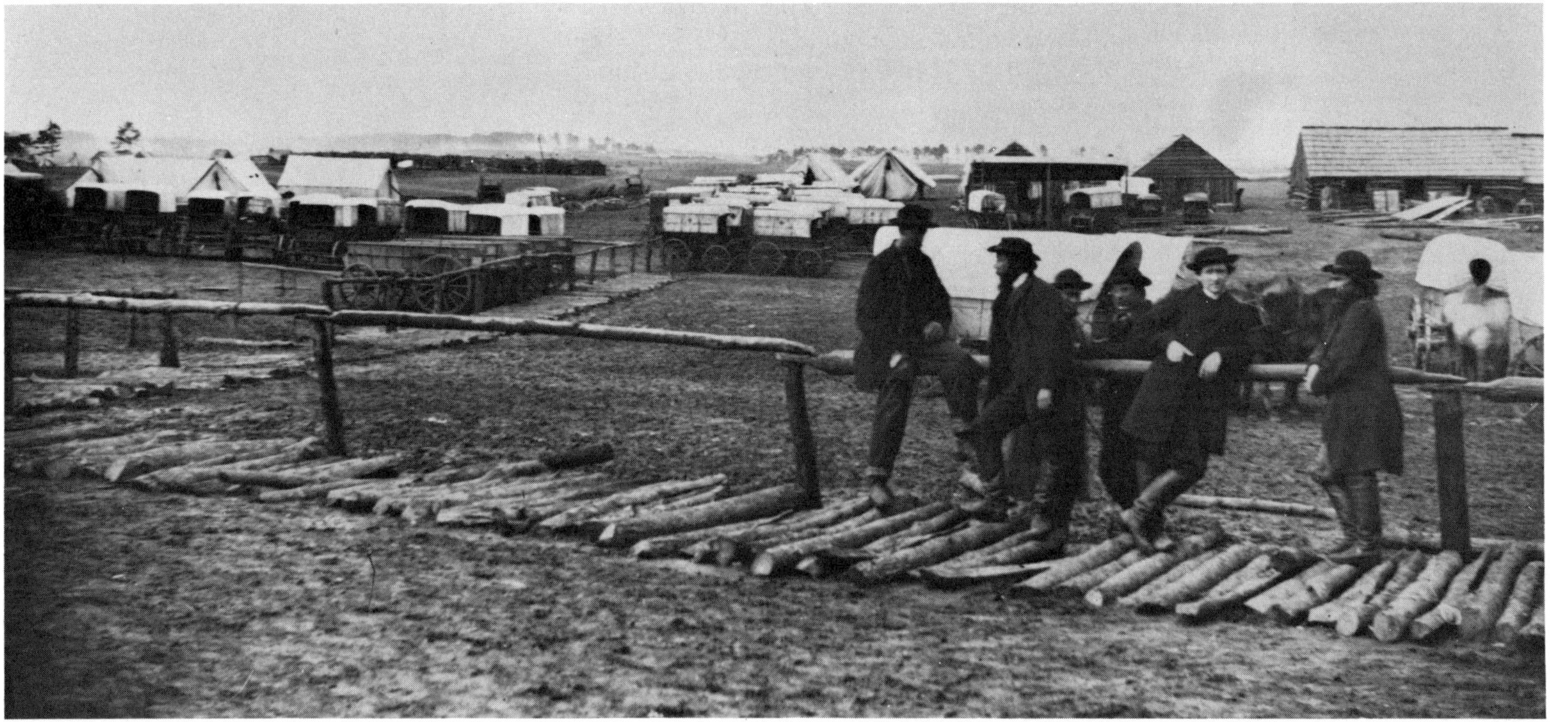

Figure 3-4, Hospital Ambulance "Corral" (Wheeler and Rucker Ambulances) *U.S. Signal Corps Brady Collection, National Archives*

and a number of assorted beer trucks and delivery vans. Civilian volunteers were added as drivers to this array of odd vehicles. But these drivers were no better than the earlier deserters. The vehicles were known to carry liquor as part of the medicinal supplies and as a consequence the disreputable drivers broke into the liquor boxes, drank the contents and immediately turned back to the safety of Washington.[12] While those who did arrive were an insolent, insubordinate, thieving lot. They stole blankets and provisions from the stores of supplies, and even a few of these craven creatures picked through the pockets of the dead and dying.[13]

Wars are heavy taskmasters—but we do learn from them. Surgeon General Hammond drew the proper deductions from the disgraceful state of affairs that existed up to the fall of 1862. He was firmly convinced that the Quartermaster's Department should not have control of the ambulances; it must be given to the Medical Department. But how? Up to now his efforts, as well as the attempts of many concerned civilian individuals and groups had been summarily ignored by the General-in-Chief, Henry W. Halleck and the Secretary of War, Edwin Stanton. Even Surgeon Tripler's proposal for a properly organized and trained ambulance corps fell on deaf ears.[14]

But as it must, in times of crises, someone appears on the scene at the crucial moment to resolve the critical situation. That was the case here. A top-notch military surgeon from the southwestern frontier had been selected to replace Surgeon Tripler as Medical Director of the Army of the Potomac. This young man was Major Jonathan Letterman. His twelve years' experience in the frontier with troops engaged in intermittent warfare against the various Indian tribes of that area had given him excellent training in the treatment, care and transportation of wounded soldiers. This, together with his administrative ability, was to prove valuable to the Army of the Potomac.[15]

Soon after reporting to General George B. McClellan, Letterman went to work. After a careful study of the deplorable battlefield conditions that plagued the Medical Department, he formulated a complete and explicit ambulance service plan for the Army of the Potomac. It is of interest to note that in all probability Surgeon Letterman was familiar with the experiences of Larrey and Percy as his plans closely resembled theirs.

General McClellan, an enthusiastic supporter of Letterman's plan, put it into effect by General Order No. 147 (August 2, 1862).[16]

In brief, the order (Letterman's Plan) specified clear and specific duties for all personnel concerned with the removal and care of the wounded troops. Continual drills and inspections were to be conducted by officers of the Medical Department. Only men of good moral character, active, efficient and interested were to be accepted for ambulance drivers and stretcher-bearers. Ambulances were to be in the *front* of all wagon trains, *and* were to be used *only* for the transportation of the sick or wounded troops. Taking a page from his European army colleagues, Letterman specified that stretcher-bearers and hospital stewards were to wear distinctive insignia on their uniforms. Paragraph fifteen of the order was long overdue and corrected an abuse that had plagued military commanders during the first two years of the war. It stated that *only* Medical Corpsmen could remove the wounded from the field of combat. The order removed one other glaring obstacle to efficient field operations by placing ambulance drivers under control of the Medical Department and by placing all ambulances, horses, harness, etc. under Division control.[17]

The favorable results of this organization became speedily apparent. At the Battle of Antietam (September 16, 1861), called the bloodiest battle of the Civil War, the ambulances of the right wing of the Union army (the left wing ambulance system was not yet operable)

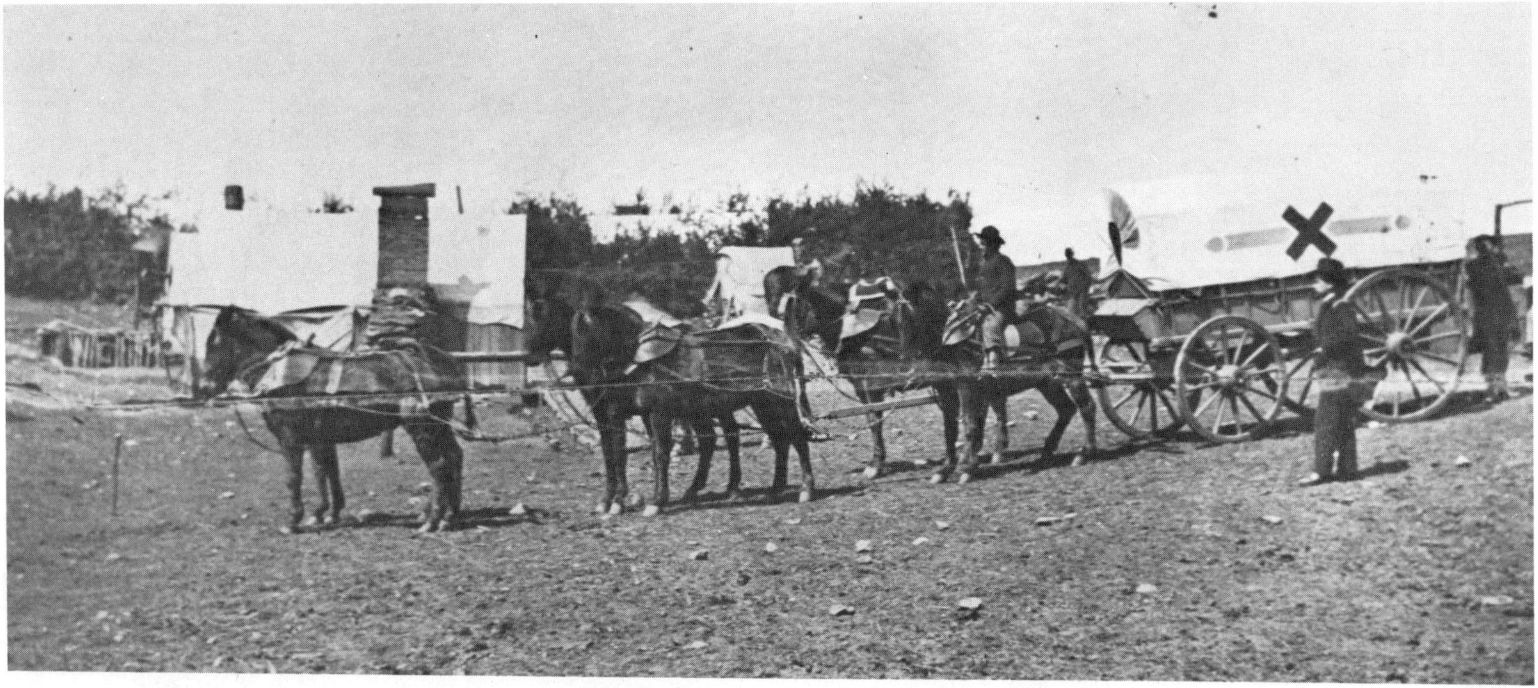

Figure 3-3, Ambulance Wagons, Sixth Corps (probably converted Army Supply Wagons) *U.S. Signal Corps Brady Collection, National Archives*

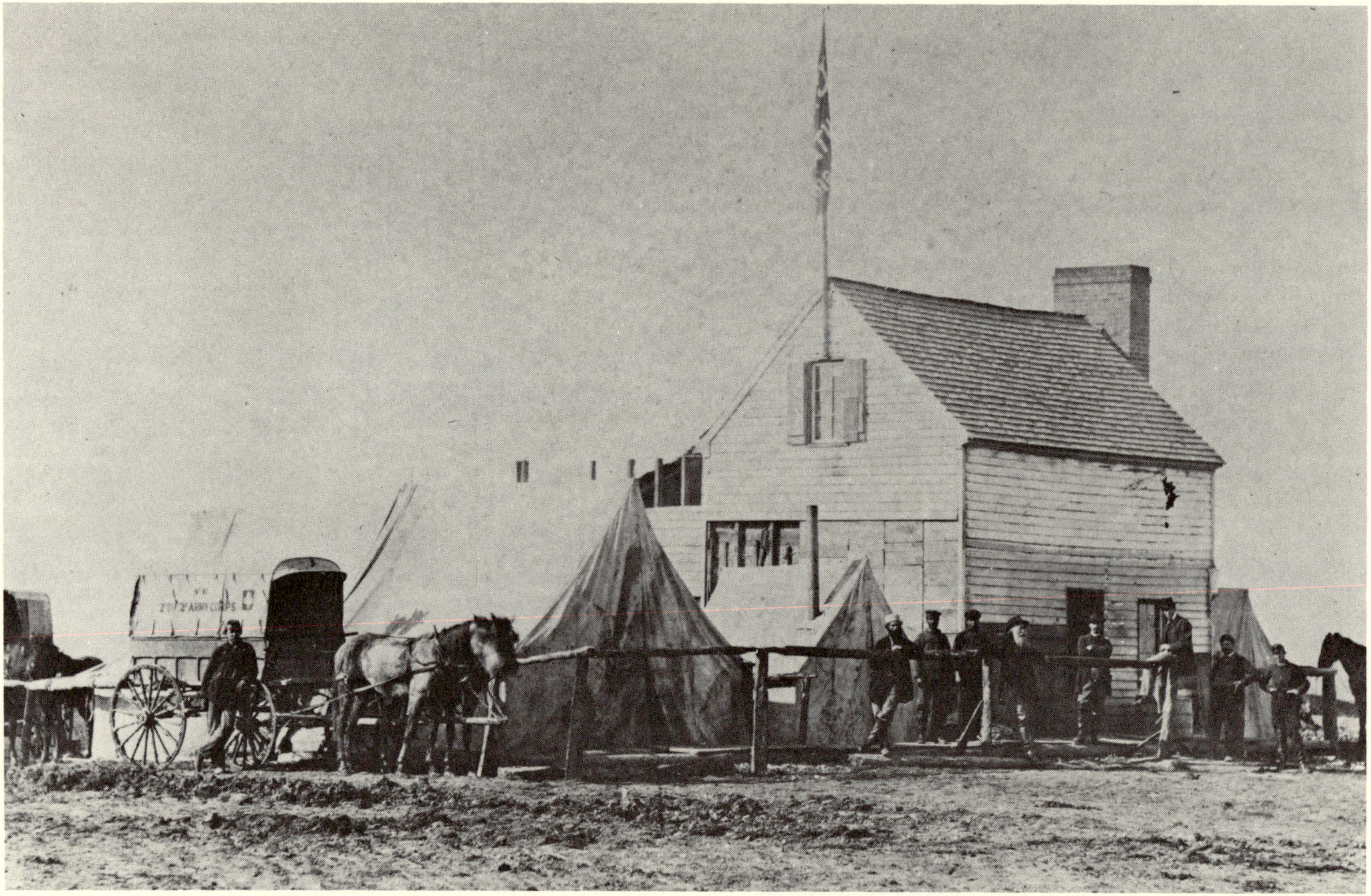

Figure 3-5, Ambulance (Rucker) in front of U.S. Sanitary Commission Headquarters. *U.S. War Dept., General Staff, National Archives*

rapidly conveyed from the combat area some 10,000 wounded soldiers. Because of the widely extended battle front (some six miles) the ambulances including the Finley two-wheelers and the cumbersome four-wheeled Triplers incessantly plied from collecting points to field hospitals. Many ambulance corpsmen proved themselves courageous beyond the call of duty when they snatched fallen comrades practically from under the muzzles of Confederate guns.[18] Again some thirty days later at Fredericksburg (December 11, 1862) the newly created ambulance corps proved so successful that the stretcherbearers and ambulances brought out the wounded faster than they could be cared for.[19]

These accomplishments of the Army of the Potomac's ambulance system so impressed Surgeon General Hammond that he (March 1863) urged all the Union armies to adopt it. This was followed on August 23, 1863 when General George C. Meade, now commander of the Army of the Potomac, issued General Order No. 85 which revised and strengthened the ambulance system.[20]

Finally after years of frustration and rebuffs from War Department officials, private civilians and professional organizations prevailed upon Congress to establish a uniform ambulance corps for the Armies of the United States. This was accomplished in the spring of 1864 when Congress passed the Act which was approved by the President on March 11, 1864. It was promulgated to the Union Armies by the Secretary of War in General Orders No. 106 (War Dept., AGO).[21] This Act followed the Letterman system almost word for word. Certainly it was a tribute to Surgeon Letterman's great ability. Unhappily the provisions of this Act would terminate upon war's end.

The effectiveness of the newly created Ambulance Corps is strikingly shown in the systematic and speedy manner with which the vast number of wounded were recovered from such gory battle sites as

Photo opposite:

Figure 3-6, A Wounded soldier lying on a Halstead Litter. *U.S. Signal Corps Brady Collection, National Archives*

the Wilderness (May 5-7, 1864), Spottsylvania (May 12, 1864), Cold Harbour (June 1-3, 1864), Petersburgh (June 15, 1864) and the campaigns in Georgia and the Carolinas right down to the war's finale on Wilmer McLean's farm at Appomatox Court House. Coincidentally it was on farmer McLean's farm near the meandering stream called Bull Run that the first battle of the Civil War took place (July 21, 1861).

Before we take leave of the countless battles, skirmishes and forays of this great conflict so hotly contested by the proud wearers of the Blue and the Gray; before we leave the chaos, the confusion and the mistakes; before the thrill of victory and the agony of defeat are forgotten, it might be well to look into the operations of the Fifth Ambulance Corps which will put in proper perspective the field operations of these dedicated men.

Here is what Captain, later Lt. Colonel, W.F. Drum reported. During May and June 1864, the Corps removed nearly 8,000 wounded in the Wilderness Campaign. It had six stretcherbearers and eight horses killed, one officer, four sergeants and seventeen stretcherbearers wounded. Owing to the severity of the fighting, thirty-four horses and twenty-six mules died. Two horses were stolen, three captured and thirty-nine horses and sixteen mules were broken down and had to be turned into the depot for rest and care. During the three days' fighting at Weldon Railroads (August 19-21, 1864), the ambulance wagons carried 773 Union and 153 Confederates to the hospital. All of this was through a heavy down-pour which turned the roads into a veritable quagmire. Here two sergeants were killed, one sergeant and five stretcherbearers wounded, nineteen stretchermen taken prisoner, eight horses killed and several ambulance wagons damaged by enemy fire. Captain Drum proudly reported that all corpsmen performed their duties faithfully and meritoriously under the greatest danger.

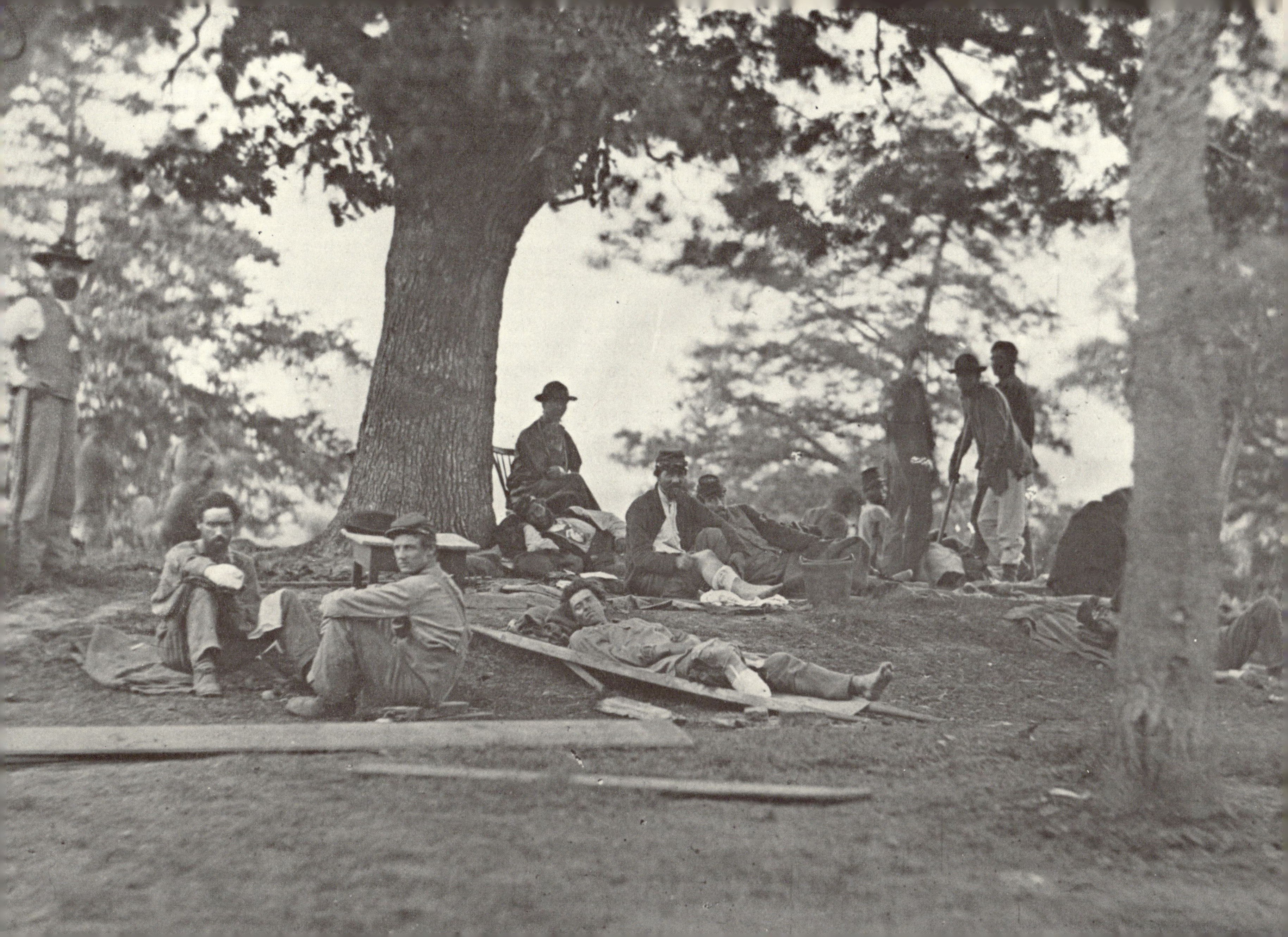

Ambulances that broke down on the march would be pulled out of line, repaired in a few minutes and returned to the march. An ambulance damaged beyond repair would be dismantled and its usable parts tied to another ambulance for future use. Only four ambulances broke down, however, during the months of May-June, 1864.[22]

Again a few extracts from the ambulance corps of Griffin's Division (First) at Fredericksburg will further show the day to day activities of the ambulance corps.

> December 11. Inspection at sunrise; teams harnessed; left camp and followed ammunition trains toward front. At sunset unhitched, but left teams harnessed all night.
>
> December 12. Hitched up at sunrise; followed ammunition trains to front; unhitched at sunset.
>
> December 13. Hitched up at sunrise; at 2 P.M. went to pontoon bridge; at 3:30 detached my stretchermen with 43 stretchers (18 regiments) and sent them across the river to the field. Detailed 12 ambulances to remain on the north side of the bridge and await the return of the stretchermen. The stretchermen were employed until 7 P.M. in bringing the wounded from the field into the city of Fredericksburg. At 7 the ambulances crossed the river, went onto the field, and were employed all night in bringing off wounded. I calculated that about 375 were removed from the field to the town that night. At 5:30 A.M. the train recrossed the river and unhitched. (This division had 665 wounded.)
>
> December 14. Remained quiet all day. Hitched up at sunrise and unhitched at sunset.
>
> December 15. Hitched up at sunrise. My train crossed the river at 10 A.M., loaded with all the wounded belonging to the division, and brought them back to this side.—Lt. Joseph C. Ayer, 18th Mass. Inf., Chief of Ambulance Corps, 1st Division, 5th Army Corps.[23]

Six months later we find Lt. Ayers and his ambulance corps at a pleasant farmland setting in southern Pennsylvania called Gettysburg.

A fair sample of the work of the ambulance corps is afforded by the report of First Lieut. Joseph C. Ayer, of the First Division, Fifth Corps, which is here given in a condensed form, with a few explanations in parentheses:

As soon as the division was placed in position all my stretcher men, under their lieutenants and sergeants, were sent to the front to follow their respective regiments; leaving one lieutenant and three sergeants in charge of the train. I conducted the train to a point two hundred yards in rear of the second and third brigades, where it was rapidly loaded with severely wounded. Owing to some misunderstanding there was a delay in locating the division hospital and the wounded men remained in the ambulances about an hour, when the hospital was established and the wounded unloaded. The ambulances then commenced regular trips to the battlefield and were constantly at work during the night.

As soon as all the wounded were secured, orders came to me to remove all the wounded in the field hospital to one farther in the rear. (The hospitals of this corps were moved on July 3d.) Previous to this, seventeen ambulances from my train had been ordered to report to the hospital of the Second Division, Fifth Corps, where they loaded with wounded, whom they conveyed to the rear. The whole of July 3d was consumed in removing the hospital. At sunset the horses were unharnessed for the first time in sixty hours.

At about 10 p.m. an order came to me to send up my whole train to the front, to remove from the field the remaining wounded of the division. On reaching the field we found but one wounded man of the Fifth Corps, but there being a sufficient number of wounded of the Third Corps, I loaded my train with them and transported them to their respective hospitals. (These were wounded of Sickles' Corps, left in the enemy's hands on the 2d. but recovered by McCandless' advance on the evening of the 3d.)

The train returned to camp near sunrise on the 4th. Having unhitched and fed, I hitched up again at 9 and reported to the several corps and division hospitals of the army, and collected as nearly as possible all wounded men of this division who had been taken to other hospitals.

On July 5th the ambulance corps received orders to move and follow the division towards Emmitsburg, leaving two ambulances and four men at the division hospital (left behind).

I estimate the total number of wounded removed from the field by the corps (First Division) to have been 560; of the Third Corps, 82. There might also be added 430 transported from one hospital to another, 53 for the Second Division, and 32 collected from other hospitals; total, 1,157, on July 2d, 3d and 4th.

The Fifth Corps, with about thirty-five regiments, some of which were battalions, had eighty-one ambulances. The wounded of this corps, 1,611 in number, were scattered over the slopes of Round Top and as far forward as the Wheatfield. The ambulances went to work at 4 p.m. on the 2d, carrying the wounded to the hospitals in rear of Little Round Top. At 4 next morning the work was complete; thirteen hundred wounded had been collected, beside some for other corps.[24]

Why the operations of this and other splendid ambulance corps are only sparingly mentioned, if at all, in the reports of general officers is hard to realize. Indeed one might read the reports of line officers, too, without knowing that the Army had either field hospitals or ambulances.

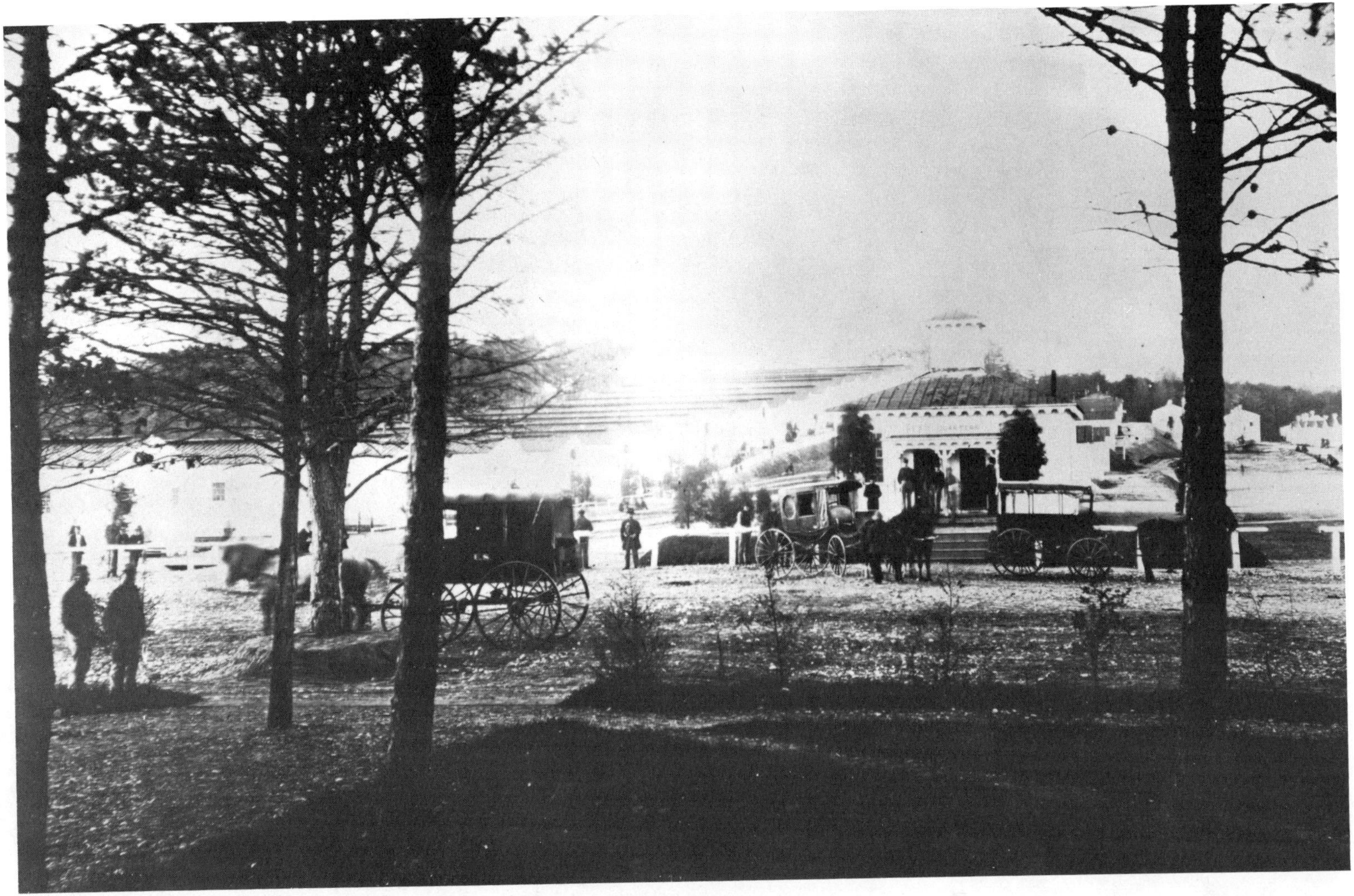

Figure 3-7, Convalescent camp, Alexandria, Virginia (note ambulance wagons left foreground, right background, probably Ruckers.
U.S. Signal Corps Brady Collection, National Archives

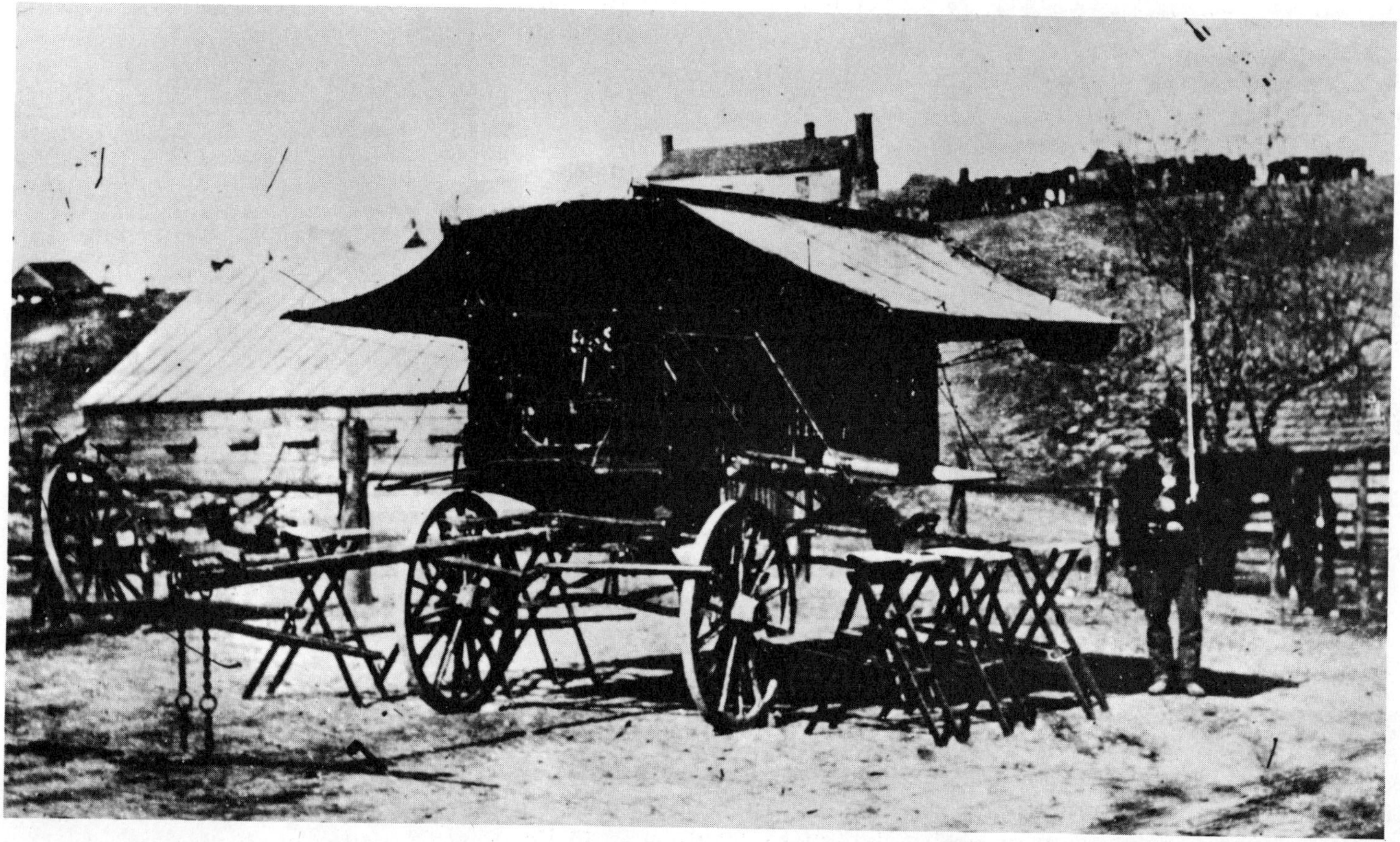

Figure 3-8, Field pharmacy - General Thomas Headquarters. *U.S. Signal Corps Brady Collection, National Archives*

Now that the last stretcherbearers have borne their pitiful burdens. Now that the bugles have sounded recall; and now that the once menacing guns have been silenced and the ceaseless tread of marching feet has been stayed, the battle flags are furled and the once vast armies, victor and vanquished, are disbanded, we are reminded of a line from Sir Walter Scott's *Lady of the Lake*, "Soldier Rest, they Warfare o'er."

NOTES

Chapter III

1. Harvey E. Brown, *The Medical Department of the United States Army, 1775-1873.* (Surgeon General's Office, Washington, D.C., 1873), p. 68.
2. Ibid., p. 68.
3. Typical of this man's thinking was his stern rebuff to General Sherman's suggestion that a hospital be built at Port Royal, South Carolina. His ridiculous reply was "The mild climate of South Carolina obviates the necessity for such a hospital." (Stewart Brooks, *Civil War Medicine*, p. 13.)
4. Surgeon General William A. Hammond (1828-1900) was born in Annapolis, Md., August 24, 1828. Took his medical degree from the University of the City of New York in 1849. Immediately entered the army as an assistant surgeon. Over the next ten years he served at various frontier posts. Hammond resigned from the army in 1859 to become professor of Anatomy and Surgery at the University of Maryland which post he held until re-entering the army in 1862. Appointed Surgeon General shortly after his re-

entry, Hammond introduced many reforms into the moribund medical administration. He ordered proper records be kept of the sick, wounded and dead; introduced a meaningful system for classification of disease; wrote and edited manuals relating to military hygiene and sanitation. In addition to his reforms he recommended the establishment of a permanent General Hospital in Washington, D.C., an Ambulance Corps, Army Medical Museum and Army Medical School.

Unfortunately due to his rather brusque manner, it was inevitable that he clashed with the erascible Secretary of War Stanton. While away on war business he was charged with a number of niggling offenses and dismissed from the service in August, 1864. A dozen years later, after the war, Hammond's case was reviewed, justice prevailed and Hammond was restored to the rank of Brigadier General. By this time he had become America's outstanding neurosurgeon. (P.M. Ashburn, *A History of the Medical Department of the U.S. Army,* p. 76. Stewart Brooks, *Civil War Medicine,* p. 20 and *Dictionary of American Biography,* Vol. IV. p. 210.)

5. Louis C. Duncan, *The Medical Department of the U.S. Army,* p. 76. Stewart Brooks, *Civil War Medicine,* p. 20 and *Dictionary of American Biography,* Vol. IV, p. 210.
6. George W. Adams, *Doctors In Blue,* p. 71.
7. Duncan (Pope's Campaign), p. 6.
8. *Medical and Surgical History of War of Rebellion,* Vol. I, Pt. I, Appendix p. 18. (Hereinafter referred to as OR.)
9. Horace H. Cunningham, *Doctors in Gray,* p. 119.
10. Adams, *Doctors in Blue,* p. 75.
11. Gen. Orders No. 20 (October 31, 1861) in OR, Vol. II, Pt. III, p. 932.

12. Adams, *Doctors in Blue*, p. 75.
13. Duncan (Bull Run), p. 48.
14. OR., Vol. II, Pt. III, p. 932.
15. Major Jonathan Letterman (1824-1872) was born in Washington County, Pennsylvania, December 11, 1824. He received his medical degree from Jefferson Medical College, Philadelphia in 1849 whereupon he immediately entered the army as an assistant surgeon. He served the twelve years at western and southwestern military posts. Here he acquired expert training in the care and transportation of wounded troops.

    In June, 1862, he was assigned to the Army of the Potomac, promoted to Major and Surgeon. Letterman possessed a high degree of administrative ability which he brought to bear upon the Medical Department of the Army of the Potomac. His basic plans for field hospitals and evacuation of sick and wounded troops influenced that service in every modern army of that time. Major Letterman resigned from the army December, 1864 and took up residence in San Francisco, California. He had married in 1863, and the sudden death of his wife four short years later was a crushing blow from which he never fully recovered. Consequently, the mental depression coupled with a chronic intestinal disorder kept him a semi-invalid until his death in 1872 at the young age of 48. The large military hospital at the Presidio of San Francisco was renamed Letterman General Hospital in his honor. (*Dictionary of American Biography*, Vol. XI, p. 194.)
16. OR., Vol. II, Pt. III, p. 935.
17. Ibid., pp. 935-937.
18. Ibid., p. 937.
19. Duncan (Fredericksburg), p. 14.
20. General Orders No. 85 in OR., Vol. II, Pt. III, p. 939.

21. OR., Vol. II, Pt. III, p. 941.
22. W.F. Drum, *Work With the Fifth Corps Ambulance Train,* pp. 79-85.
23. Duncan (Fredericksburg), p. 15.
24. Ibid., (Gettysburg), pp. 15-16.

Chapter Four

ON THE WESTERN INDIAN FRONTIER

"For This We Are Soldiers"
—*Gen. Guy V. Henry*

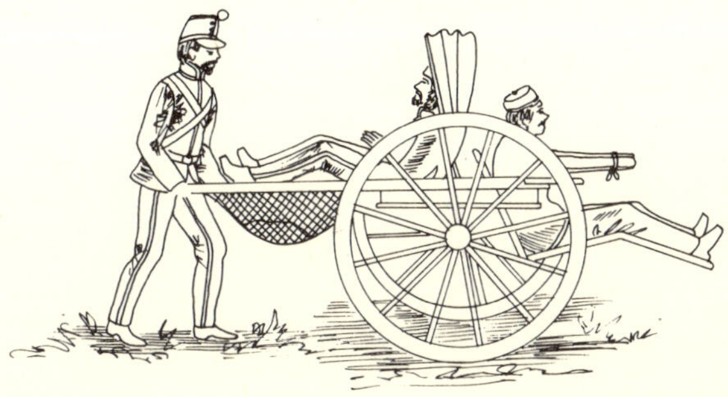

The command (1) Prepare to mount, (2) MOUNT barked in Irish brogue or guttural German rang out across the assembly area as troopers and horses, alike, impatiently waited for the command to march out. That command having been given, with guidons fluttering in the slight breeze, the troopers clattered excitedly through the main gate to confront whatever mission that might lay ahead, whether it be escort duty, guard duty or full-scale skirmish against the clever Indian foe.

The loneliness and deadly routine of garrison duty could not be forgotten in the excitement and expectation of doing that which a soldier is expected to do—fight the foe. While these encounters were always welcomed, they did have a melancholy price. One could be felled by arrow or bullet during the heat of battle, or fall silently into a deep ravine, body pierced by a silent arrow of a Sioux or Cheyenne warrior, there to lie in mortal agony until collected and transported to safety on some quickly devised conveyance.

As soon as the battle or skirmish ended and sometimes in the heat of action, soldiers did what they could for their wounded comrades. Often without the direction of a surgeon and untrained in first aid (until the late eighties), soldiers gave their wounded companions such make-shift care as limited time and material afforded. No individual first aid packets were issued during the Indian campaigns. Few rank and file regulars knew how to stop dangerous bleeding.[1] First aid advice in "The Soldier's Handbook" gave the barest minimum of instructions. An explanation that cuts healed more quickly than bullet wounds; that wounded soldiers should be placed on their backs and given a drink of water; that there were two types of bleeding, veinous and arterial, with the latter requiring a tourniquet, constituted the first aid advice.[2]

Because so many engagements against the hostile Indians frequently took place in unexplored regions, remote and inaccessible to wheeled vehicles, pack animals and man were the only means of bringing a fallen soldier to medical care.

Facilities for moving casualties, once they were carried to points where wheeled vehicles could pick them up, were woefully inadequate. Many companies and detachments had no wheeled ambulances at all, and often times those that did have a few ambulances on hand couldn't find one when needed as, in all likelihood, it was being used for private transportation. Whenever visiting dignitaries from Washington or foreign countries desired to visit military posts "out West," the light spring ambulance was furnished for their use. In fact, these vehicles became so popular for private and semi-official business, that they were often referred to as the "Quartermaster stage on the plains."

One of the most common and quickly made conveyances used by the frontier regulars was the Indian travois. This type of conveyance, according to Francis Parkman, eminent nineteenth century historian, had been used by the American colonists as early as 1763. Lewis and Clark resorted to its use in carrying the sick and wounded of their explorations. And, as a result of our many engagements against the western Indian, our military surgeons found the travois well adapted to the necessities of frontier service.[3]

Another conveyance much in use, too, was the two-horse/mule litter which was so successfully utilized by Surgeon Satterlee during the Seminole War of 1835. In fact, Army regulations (1861) authorized its use where wheeled vehicles were not practicable.[4] As a matter of fact, a survey of the literature touching upon the frontier army's transportation of its sick and wounded quite clearly indicated that the travois, the two-horse/mule litter and hand litters were the most effective conveyances in use. All three had their adherents, so let us see what a representative cross-section of the military surgeons associated with these litters has to say.

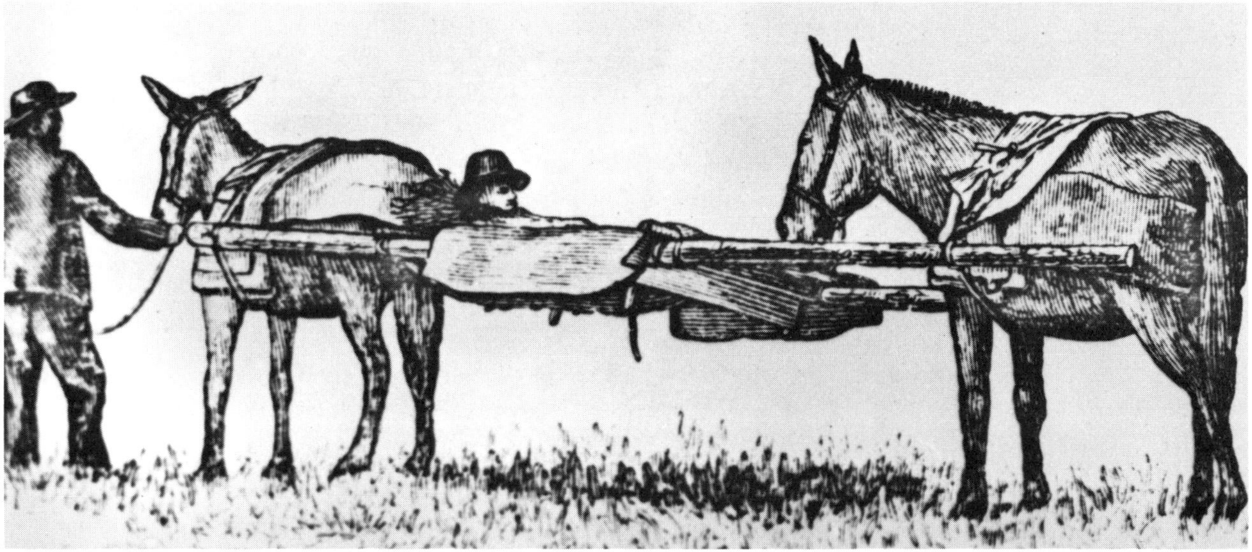

Figure 4-1, Wounded soldier conveyed on a Double-Mule Litter (Otis, S.G.O. Circular No. 9)

Assistant Surgeon Curtis E. Munn, Senior Medical Officer of General Crook's Powder River Expedition against the Sioux (March, 1876), reported that the expedition which headed north from Fort Fetterman, Wyoming Territory hadn't gone more than thirty miles from the fort when Indians fired on two herders who accompanied the troops, severly wounding one of them. Surgeon Munn had this fellow placed in one of the ambulance wagons (probably a Rucker) and taken some eighty miles to a camp on Crazy Women's Fork. Anticipating a large number of wounded from this expedition, Munn instructed one of his assistants, a civilian Dr. Ridgely, to establish a field hospital at Old Fort Reno. Dr. Ridgely's failure to fully comply with Surgeon Munn's instruction was to later result in much discomfort to the wounded soldiers that were brought in.

About one week later further along the trail, Munn had an opportunity to become well acquainted with the travois when he was obliged to place a Corporal Moore (Co. D. 3d. U.S. Cavalry) upon one of these. Corporal Moore, whose horse had fallen upon him, had a most comfortable ride of several days upon the travois. A few days later (March 17), the command struck an Indian village and after several hours of intense fighting, Private Egan (Co. K. 2d. U.S. Cavalry) received a serious wound in the abdomen. He was placed in a travois and conveyed some 100 miles over "the roughest trails to the ambulance station" with very little discomforture. The effective use of the travois in these instances was not lost upon Surgeon Munn who observed that the travois was a comfortable and safe method of transporting wounded troops and further declared "I would recommend the employment of this mode of transportation wherever troops are obliged to leave wagon roads."[5]

However, Munn's opinion was not wholly endorsed by Assistant Surgeon Albert Hartsuff, who employed both the two-horse litter and the travois after a particularly hot engagement against the Sioux in Rosebud Creek, Wyoming Territory (June 17, 1876).

As soon as the fierce fighting ended, Surgeon Hartsuff, with the aid of Mr. Moore, the Chief Packer, set about constructing travois and two-horse litters. Colonel Guy V. Henry, 3d. U.S. Cavalry, the most seriously wounded (shattered jaw)[6] was carefully placed on one of the horse litters, five of the other badly wounded soldiers rode the travois, while thirteen of the less severely wounded rode their own horses. Commenting on the types of conveyances used by this little cavalcade of casualties, Hartsuff said, "I carefully watched the behavior of the litter and the travois. I soon discovered, however, that the two-horse litter was much better in all respects than the travois, except, perhaps, over comparatively smooth ground..."[7]

Many wounded soldiers of the Indian Fighting Army, though, were in circumstances where they couldn't take advantage of the travois or the two-horse litter. One such hapless fellow while fighting the Modocs at Lava Beds (January 18, 1873) had the misfortune to have an artery severed and was not expected to live. Four of his comrades placed him in a blanket litter to carry him to an aid station thirteen nightmarish hours distant. And, as if that weren't enough torture, the luckless soldier had to ride a jolting army wagon some thirty miles further to the nearest military hospital at Fort Klamath.[8] So far as is known, this man survived his ordeal.

Military surgeons of the Indian Fighting Army, in addition to professional ability, had to be masters of improvisation. Witness the predicament of Surgeon James Kimball. During the Yellowstone Expedition (August, 1873), organized to protect the party surveying the route of the Northern Pacific Railway and to select new sites for army posts, a Lieutenant Charles Braden, Seventh U.S. Cavalry, and his men came under intense fire from a large body of Sioux. Lieutenant

Braden was felled by a bullet through his thigh bone which became progressively worse by the jolting of the army ambulance over the rough prairie to such an extent that the half-crazed officer begged Surgeon Kimball to dispatch him then and there. Instead, Kimball cooly surveyed the situation and devised, on the spot, a new style litter—a canvas stretcher hung between two sets of wheels drawn by the seemingly ever-faithful, ever-present army mule. On this speedily improvised conveyance, the wounded officer was transported in grand style to a military hospital several hundred miles away—and lived to tell the story.[9]

Don Rickey, Jr., in his definitive study of the daily lives of the frontier regulars, *Forty Miles a Day On Beans and Hay,* relates an amusing incident that involved a travois, a wounded soldier and a fractious mule which occurred shortly after the Dull Knife Fight (November 25, 1876). It seems that the mule pulling the travois became unruly. While Lieutenant Wheeler was reprimanding the Corporal in charge of the travois, the wounded soldier on the travois cried out, "Let 'er go Lieutenant. If I had sleigh bells, I'd think I was taking a sleigh ride." In spite of a serious hip wound, this light-hearted soldier made the journey to the hospital in comfort. But not so another disabled soldier who begged, "Make this [travois] easier for me or kill me to get me out of my misery."[10]

From *Forty Miles a Day on Beans and Hay: The Enlisted Soldier Fighting the Indian Wars,* by Don Rickey, Jr. Copyright 1963 by the University of Oklahoma Press.

Tuesday morning, June 27th, 1876, dawned warm and slightly hazy as members of Lieutenant Edward Godfrey's command (Co. K) enjoyed the pleasure of a square meal without the rattle of gunfire when a cloud of dust was observed several miles down river. Fearing a return of the Indian warriors, assembly was sounded, horses moved to protection, camp kettles and canteens filled with water, all in readiness should there be a renewal of the fight of the day before. Sixty suspense-filled minutes agonizingly ticked away until the cloud of dust

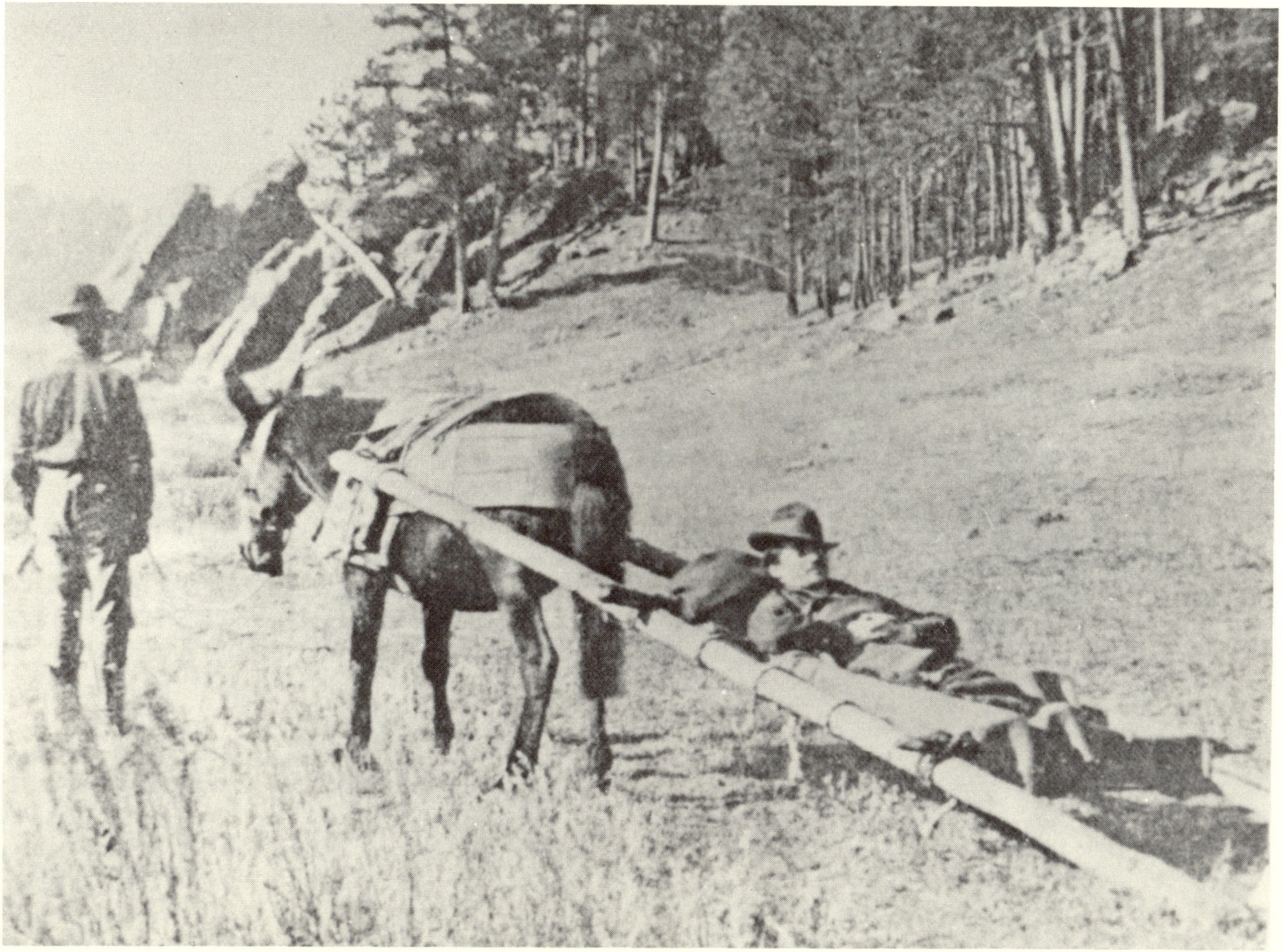

Figure 4-2a, Wounded man - General Crook's Command, Transported by Travois, 1876
(Rickey, *Forty Miles a Day on Beans and Hay,* Permission University of Oklahoma Press, Norman)

resolved itself into the person of Lieutenant James Bradley (Seventh U.S. Infantry). He had come to announce the tragic news that General Custer's immediate command had been annihilated.[11] Generals Terry and Gibbon, with their commands, arrived soon after, whereupon the grisly tasks of burial and collection of the wounded got underway.

Surgeons John Williams and Holmes O. Paulding of General Terry's command hastened to Major Reno's position on the bluffs where they quickly came to the aid of the exhausted Dr. Henry Porter. This dedicated surgeon had labored unceasingly and alone through two harrowing days and nights, often under intense enemy fire to administer to the wounded and dying of Reno's command.

It was urgent that the wounded be moved immediately to the army transport "Far West" lying at anchor some thirty miles away. General Gibbon suggested hand stretchers, Surgeon Williams travois, while Lieutenant Doane (2d. U.S. Cavalry) advocated the two-horse litters. All three were made and used in moving five miles down the Little Big Horn to a cleaner and less cluttered area.

This initial move of some six hours was accompanied by utter confusion, frustration and the complete discomfort of many of the wounded who were carried on the hand litters. They proved useless. The travois worked well. Except for luggage, the two-horse litters didn't work so well due to the restless, jittery animals. Many of the wounded feared to be placed on the two-horse litters.[12]

Next morning new attempts were made to improve the transportation situation. The hand litters were discarded. More travois and mule litters were made. Lieutenant Doane took charge; he was still confident that his mule litters would work, so he set his men to constructing them while he selected animals from General Custer's pack train as being more docile and tractable. By 5 p.m. the column with its grim burden of wounded recommenced its melancholy journey to the

"Far West." The more seriously wounded, including Private Michael Madden (Co. K, amputated leg), were placed on the two-mule litters, ten on travois and thirty of the less wounded rode their horses. Each mule litter was attended by four men to assure complete comfort to the patient. One of the men led the forward mule, one the rear mule, while the two others walked on either side of the litter to keep it steady. Only one little mishap occurred as the train neared the "Far West," the leading mule of Private Madden's litter knelt down, rolling him off onto the ground, but he was not seriously hurt.[13]

The march of mercy ended shortly after midnight, June 30th, and by dawn of the following day, the long-suffering wounded were safely bedded down on the hay strewn decks of the "Far West."[14]

The Travois

A conveyance that transports sick and wounded in which one end rests on the ground, the other end secured to the animal drawing it. In its simplest form, it consists of two poles, sixteen to seventeen feet long, four to six inches in diameter, with crossbars approximately thirty inches long attached to the two poles to keep them rigid. A piece of canvas, animal hide or other suitable material is attached to the poles and cross pieces to form a bed for the patient. This type of conveyance can be made on the spot in fifteen minutes or so providing the necessary materials are at hand.

This type of conveyance had been used by the Indians for centuries to transport baggage, children, and sick and ailing relatives. The early American Colonists resorted to its use on many occasions, and Lewis and Clark called it into service whenever they had to transport sick or injured members of their westward expedition in 1804-1806.

The field service of these primitive conveyances has been proven time and time again. Practically all the military surgeons familiar with their use have praised them for their simple and easy construction, for their ability to move in narrow places, and for the comfort accorded the patients in riding them.

Assistant Surgeon Julius H. Patzki remarked that the military surgeon could always rely on the "old traditional travois" which can ordinarily be constructed on the spot.[1]

On returning from the Powder River Expedition against the Sioux in the winter of 1876, Assistant Surgeon J.R. Gibbon related that the traditional travois with its rude construction and apparent imperfections, was in reality a great boon to the conveyance of casualties.

As it happens with any type of product, someone comes along with an idea for its improvement. The travois was not immune from some tinkering. Several of the military surgeons made efforts to standardize this conveyance. Needless to say, all the proposed models merely added some special appurtenances to the simple Indian model.

Assistant Surgeon Peter A.J. Cleary proposed that each side pole which forms the shafts be jointed and held in place by an easily removable pin so that the travois could be used as a hand stretcher when that need arose. All dimensions of his travois were comparable to the originals. One feature of interest about Surgeon Cleary's litter, though, was not the litter itself, but the harness. In addition to the regular girth to which the poles were attached, Cleary added a hip strap to pass over the horses's hips and be attached to the shafts of the travois in such a manner that the litter could not be upset should the horse rear up or kick about.

Surgeon Charles Greenleaf proposed a travois similar to Cleary's. The shafts held together by a collar arrangement could be separated when a hand stretcher needed to be used.

Nevertheless, none of these proposed models were ever adopted by the U.S. Army. It was content to use the old traditional Indian travois which met the test of time in grand style.

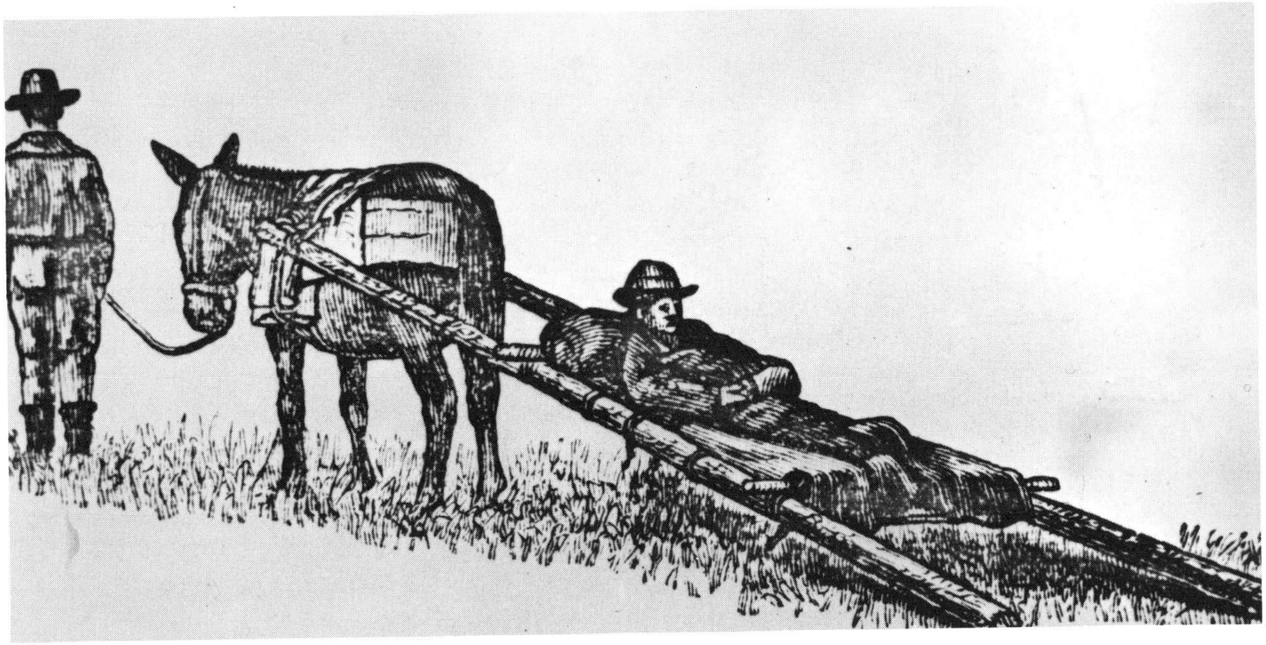

Figure 4-2, Wounded soldier on a Travail or Travois (Otis, S.G.O. Circular No. 9)

NOTES

Chapter IV

1. Rickey, Don, Jr., *Forty Miles A Day on Beans and Hay,* University of Oklahoma Press, Norman (1963), p. 323.
2. Hershler, N., *The Soldier's Handbook,* Government Printing Office, Washington, D.C. (1884), p. 52-54.
3. Otis, George A., "Transportation of the Sick and Wounded by Pack Animal." *War Department, Surgeon's General Office, Circular No. 9* (1877), p. 17.
4. War Department, Army Regulations, 1861 (Revised), par. 1298.
5. Otis, p. 19.
6. Colonel Guy V. Henry, West Point, class of 1856, recovered from his serious wounds. For his gallentry at Rosebud Creek, he was promoted to Brigadier General and went on to serve his nation honorably and faithfully until retirement in June, 1899. (Heitman, Francis B., *Historical Record of the U.S. Army, 1783-1903,* 2 vols., Washington, D.C. (1903).
7. Otis, p. 20.
8. Miller, Colonel William H., "Incidents of the Modoc War," quoted in Rickey, p. 326.
9. Kimball, Maria B., *A Soldier Doctor of Our Army,* Houghton-Mifflin, Boston (1917), p. 69.
10. Rickey, p. 328.
11. Graham, Colonel W.A., *The Custer Myth,* Bonanza Books, New York City (1953), p. 146.
12. Otis, p. 23.
13. Otis, p. 23.
14. Lieutenant Gustavus C. Doane, 3rd U.S. Cavalry, one of the unsung heroes of the Little Big Horn Battle, rose to rank of Captain, 1884. Died May 5, 1892.

For his energy and skill in providing for this transportation of the wounded to the steamer "Far West," he received high commendation from both Generals Terry and Gibbon. General Alfred Terry, in his report to the Assistant Adjutant General, Division of the Missouri (December 7, 1876), praised Lieutenant Doane in these words, "...I feel the most hearty admiration for the zeal, skill and energy displayed by this accomplished gentleman and soldier."

General Gibbon of the 7th U.S. Infantry, in an endorsement to the Adjutant General of the Department of the Dakotas (July 18, 1876), invited the attention of the Department Commander to the highly valuable service of Lieutenant Doane in these words, "But for his energy, skill and perserverance, our suffering wounded would all probably have remained exposed for several days longer in the field."

(Both of the above communications are quoted from Adjutant General Office, Consolidated Correspondence File, Letters Received, R.G. 94, Entry 622, National Archives.)

Chapter Five

LITTERS, CACOLETS & AMBULANCE WAGONS

litters, cacolets and ambulance wagons

In which are examined the specifications, construction, description, cost and field service of conveyances used to transport wounded troops in the Civil War and in the numerous forays against hostile Indians from the swamps of Florida westward to the shores of the Pacific.

SECTION ONE

Litters Borne by Man

The first removal of the wounded from the battlefield was generally by hand litter. These litters of one pattern or another are as old as warfare itself.

Probably the very first type of litter borne by man was a seat fashioned by two men grasping each others wrists in such a way as to form a seat for the patient. This litter could carry a person only until the bearers' hands and wrists gave out. Then, too, only slightly wounded men could be carried in this manner. Seriously wounded soldiers who were forced to be carried in a recumbent position would have to be taken in a blanket or canvas litter.

Blankets held at each of the four corners by the four bearers were often employed to carry seriously wounded comrades. The disadvantage of this litter was the difficulty in keeping it taut enough. Too often, the patient would soon assume a folded or slumped position, and this could prove fatal to victims of chest, abdomen and hip wounds. Besides, four men to carry one wounded comrade was an uneconomical use of manpower. Muskets were often used as stretcher poles to give some rigidity to the blanket, but then this type of litter was hard to carry because the muskets were not long enough to allow for a proper walking stride.

Sashes, too, were often times used by early European fighting men. You no doubt have seen pictures of these gentlemen, officers and noncommissioned officers, decked out with sashes. It might be of interest to note that they were actually issued these sashes to be used to convey them from the battlefield should they or their comrades become wounded in the struggle. The halberds or halberts, the seven-foot, spear-battleaxes, were used as poles in the sashes.[1] Other improvised litters of this general type could be, and probably were, devised on the spot. One was a hammock-like affair slung under a pole, either end of the pole placed in the bearers' shoulders. All of these litters had two great disadvantages: (1) they all sagged with the weight of the patient causing him some discomfort, and (2) they were rather cumbersome and awkward for the bearers to carry any distance.

As the centuries passed and the equipment of warfare became more organized and sophisticated, improvements were noted in the transportation of the sick and wounded soldiers. Litters to be borne by men were manufactured and issued to the troops as part of their regular impedimenta. During the Civil War years which saw our first efforts toward organized casualty removal, the Property Division of the Surgeon General's Office showed that over 52,000 hand litters or stretchers of various models were purchased and issued to the Union troops between 1861 and 1865.[2]

The Satterlee

At the beginning of the Civil War, the Satterlee, or U.S. Regulation litter, designed by Surgeon R.S. Satterlee, was supplied to all the regiments. Specifications of this litter are:

Poles - Seasoned red ash, 8'9" long, 1½" diameter.

Canvas Bed - Two pieces of canvas, 5'10" long, 27" wide, sewed in the center with a flat seam. A hem 7½" wide was

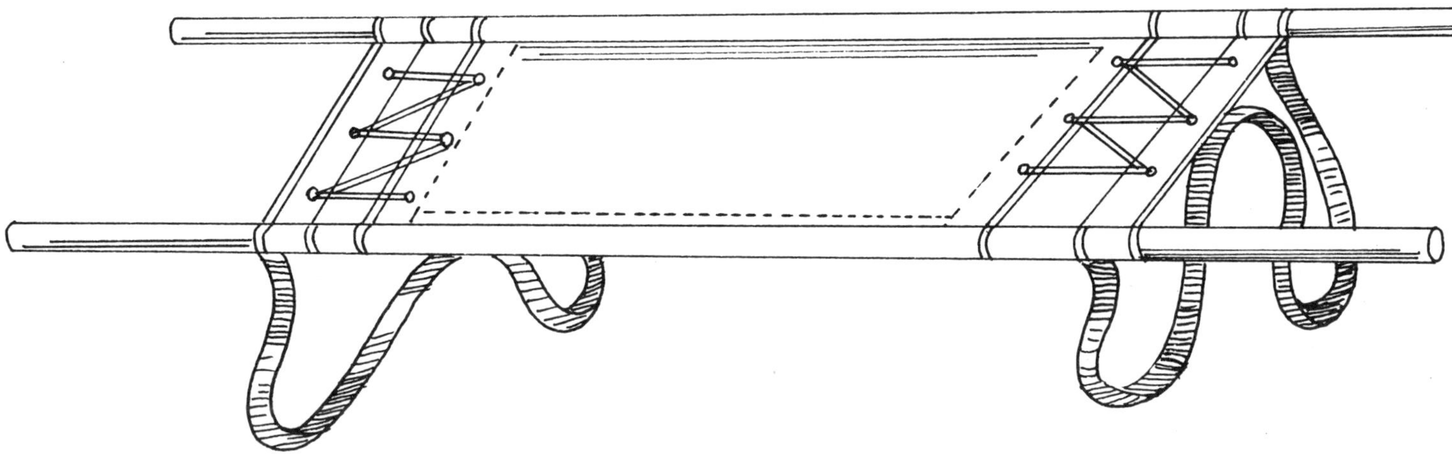

Figure 5-1, Satterlee or Regulation U.S. Army Litter
Redrawn from *Medical Surgical History, War of Rebellion,* Part III, Vol. II

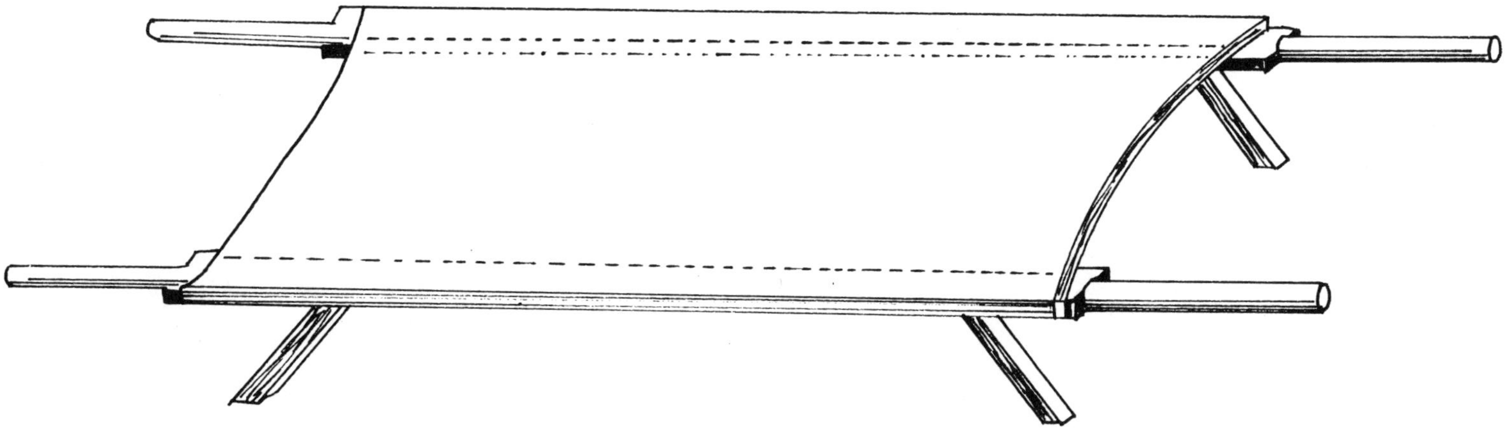

Figure 5-2, Halstead's Litter
Redrawn from *Medical-Surgical History, War of Rebellion,* Part III, Vol. II

sewed on either side of the canvas through which the poles were passed. The canvas was fastened to crossbars at either end by strong tarred ropes passed through metal eyelets.

Crossbars - Seasoned white ash, 24" long, 1½" in diameter.

Legs - A 6' piece of wrought iron, 1" wide by ¼" thick, was fashioned and fastened to the underside of the poles to form legs for the litter.

Straps - Adjustable leather straps were provided so that the bearers could ease the weight of the load if they so desired.

Weight - 24½ pounds.[3]

One of the chief objections to the Satterlee was its bulk which seriously interfered with its portability. Although replaced to some extent by other stretcher patterns, it could be found in many ambulance trains, even finding its way to the Indian frontier where it was in use for many, many years.

Although ample references to the number of stretchers issued to the regiments have been found, nothing was seen regarding manufacturer or cost.

The Halstead

As it happens in all times of national emergencies, certain persons motivated by patriotism or deep concern for humanity devise, design and place at the government's doorstep certain creations of their minds and ingenuity. So it was with hand litters. One such was a person by the name of Halstead who came forth with a light compact stretcher which soon gained much favor with the medical personnel and soon superseded the Satterlee. Specifications of this litter are:

Poles - White ash, 8' long, 1-5/16" square, rounded off at

the ends to form easily grasped handles.

Canvas Bed - 5'11" long, 23" wide, fastened to the poles by 6-ounce tacks.

Crossbars - None. Iron braces at either end held the stretcher open. These braces were hinged in the center so that the stretcher could be closed when not in use. When open, the hinged braces shut in a pin-and-bolt arrangement which prevented it from accidentally closing.

Legs - Four legs of seasoned white oak, 14" long, 1-7/8" wide at top, tapering to 1-3/8" at the bottom. They were attached to the poles by means of screw bolts.

Straps - Adjustable shoulder straps of cotton webbing with leather ends were provided should the bearers decide to use them.

Pillow - A canvas-covered hair pillow was also provided.

Weight - 23-3/4 pounds.

While this litter was reported to have given satisfactory service, it proved too fragile for hard usage. 12,867 of these were issued out of the Medical Purveyor's Depot, New York City.[4]

The Schell

Another hand litter similar in design to the Halstead was designed by Assistant Surgeon Henry S. Schell.

The main feature of Schell's litter was that it could be used as a bedstead, if necessary. The ends of the side poles were hinged and could be turned down to form the legs of the bed. These legs were held in place by strong iron stays.[5]

Two chief objections to this litter, which could well include the

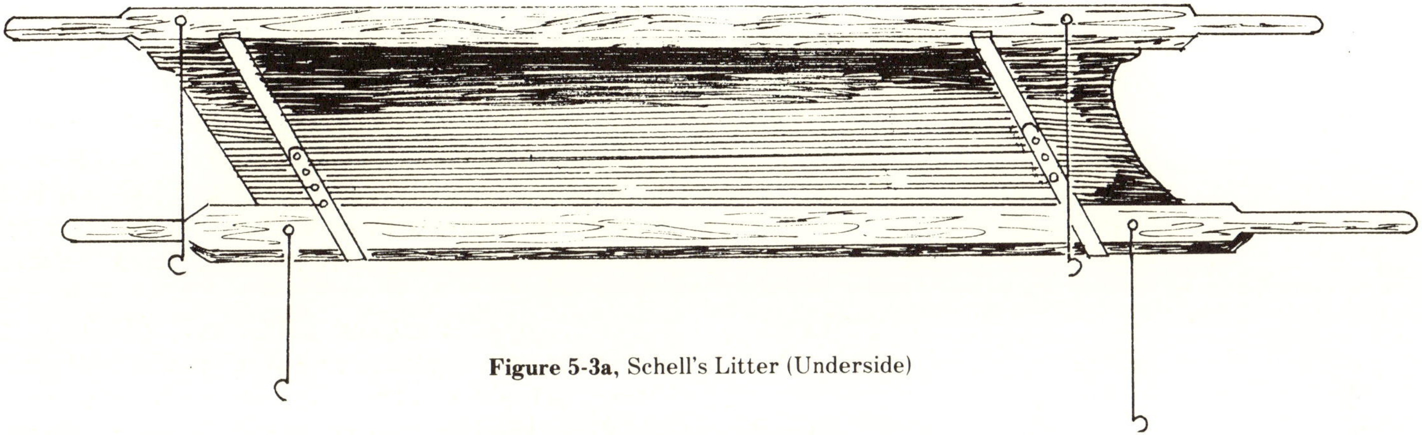

Figure 5-3a, Schell's Litter (Underside)

Figure 5-3b, Schell's Litter (Used as a cot)
Redrawn from *Medical-Surgical History, War of Rebellion,* Part III, Vol. II

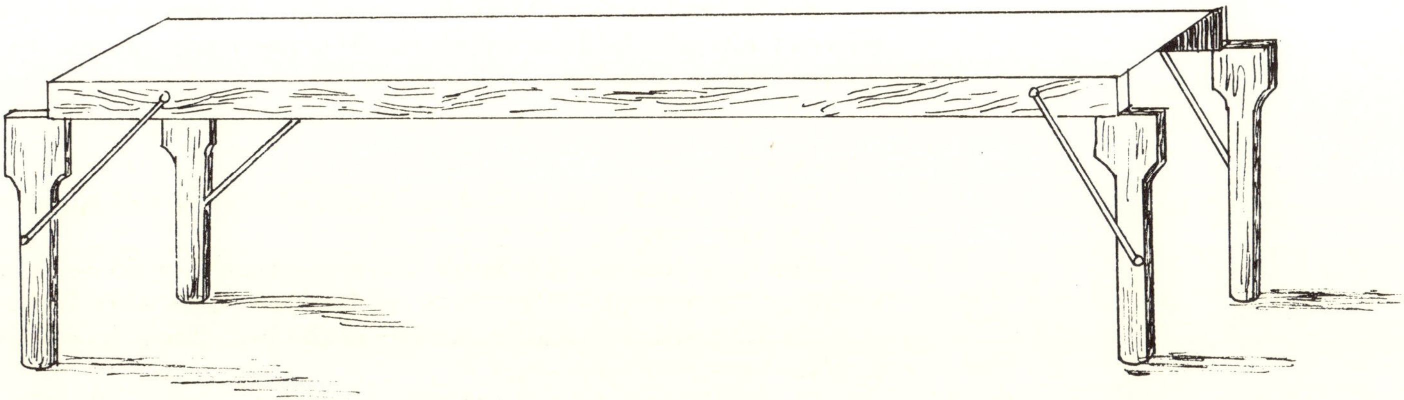

Halstead, were that the bearers would need extra help to set the legs for lowering it to the ground, and the legs could be easily broken off.

There were a few reports, too, that officers used these litters for cots, and were indignant when forced to give them up.

The United States Sanitary Commission designed a light-weight, compact litter which proved too fragile for hard usage in the tough-going of actual combat.

Before concluding this section, it might be well to point out that the stretcher bearers should have an aptitude for handling wounded personnel. They should, in fact, have all the requisites of hospital stewards. When working in pairs, the bearers should be very nearly the same height and weight. In walking with the stretcher, they must walk evenly with a light, springy step and be sure to keep the stretcher level with the ground at all times.

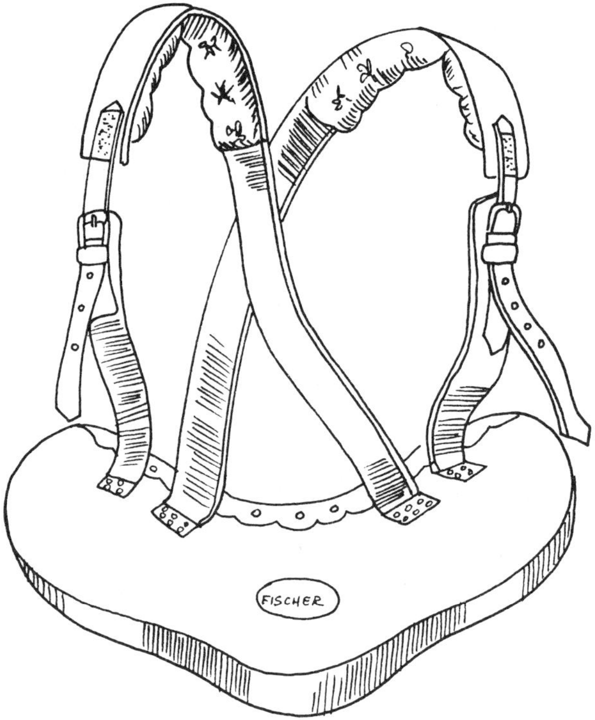

Figure 5-4, Fischer's Apparatus for Carriage of Wounded Men on Bearers Back (European model)
Redrawn from Longmore's *Treatise on Wounded Troops, 1866*

Figure 5-5, Turner's Tent Hammock used as hand litter (European model) Redrawn from Longmore's *Treatise, 1866*

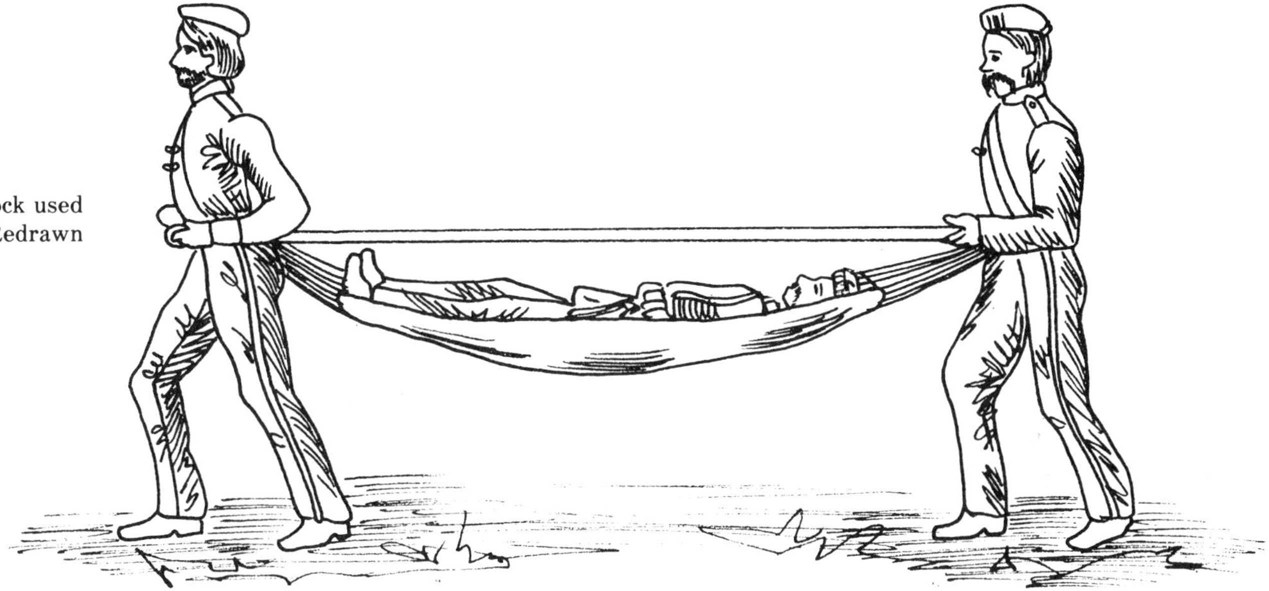

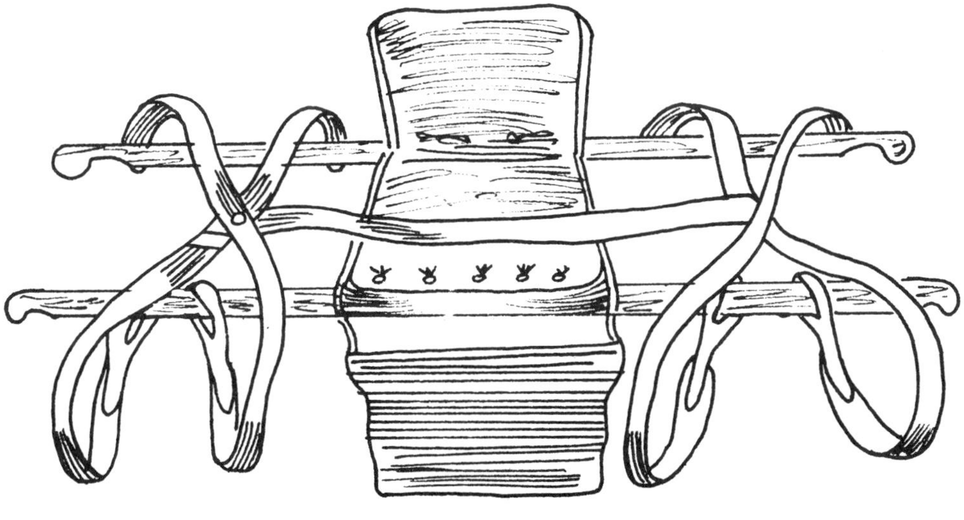

Figure 5-6, Cacolet or Chair Stretcher for Carriage by two bearers abreast or in file (European model)
Redrawn from Longmore's *Treatise, 1866*

SECTION TWO

Litters Wheeled by Man

While there was no reported use of this type of conveyance by the U.S. Army, the Index of U.S. Patents, Volume I, listed a Mr. C.H. Tompkins as receiving a patent, number 57,013, on August 27, 1866. Unfortunately, this patent drawing was missing from the files. One report did have it that Tompkins litter was simply a wheeled stretcher with canopy and protective covering for the patient, attached similarly to the ones so successfully used in the Danish War of 1864.[1]

Probably the only type of wheeled vehicle used by U.S. troops was the humble, simple wheelbarrow pressed into use by our Revolutionary War forefathers. This undistinguished conveyance was repeatedly used as ambulance transportation in the European battle fronts.

Larrey, the great and gifted military surgeon of Napoleon's armies in his account of the Russian campaign related that after the Battle of Bautzen in Saxony (summer, 1813), two-thirds of the wounded were transported to Dresden, some thirty miles distant. Larrey added that he had seen as many as 150 wheelbarrows in single file on the road from Bautzen to Dresden.[2]

This particular type of wheelbarrow was in general use in the country to carry provisions and merchandise. The peculiar shape of the wheelbarrow so fitted the contours of a person's body that he could ride quite comfortably in this unpretentious conveyance.

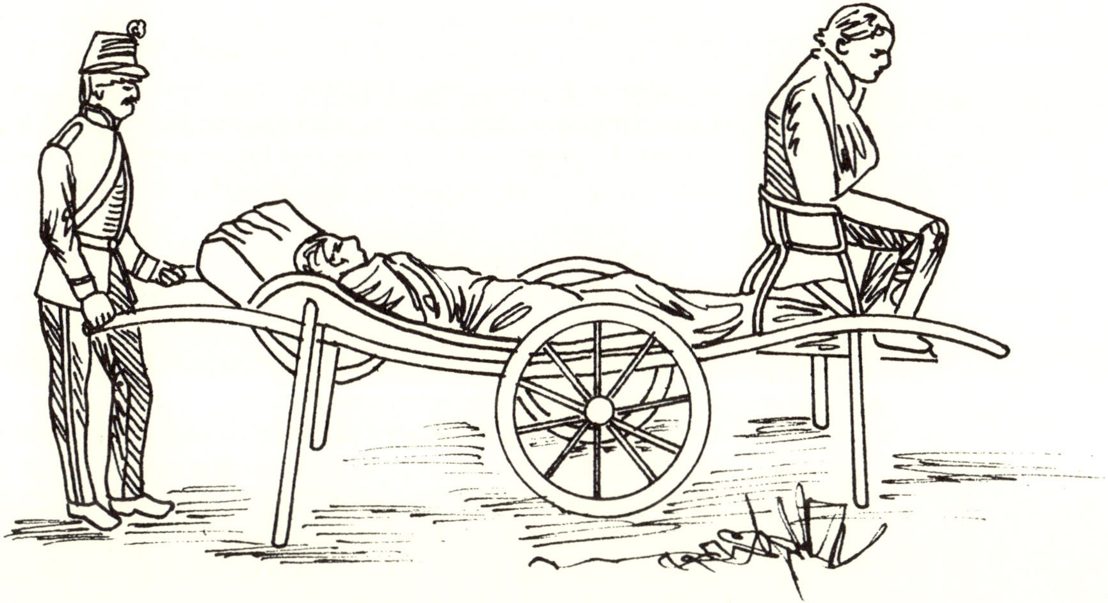

Figure 5-7, Evan's Hand-Wheeled Litter (European model)
Redrawn from Longmore's *Treatise, 1866*

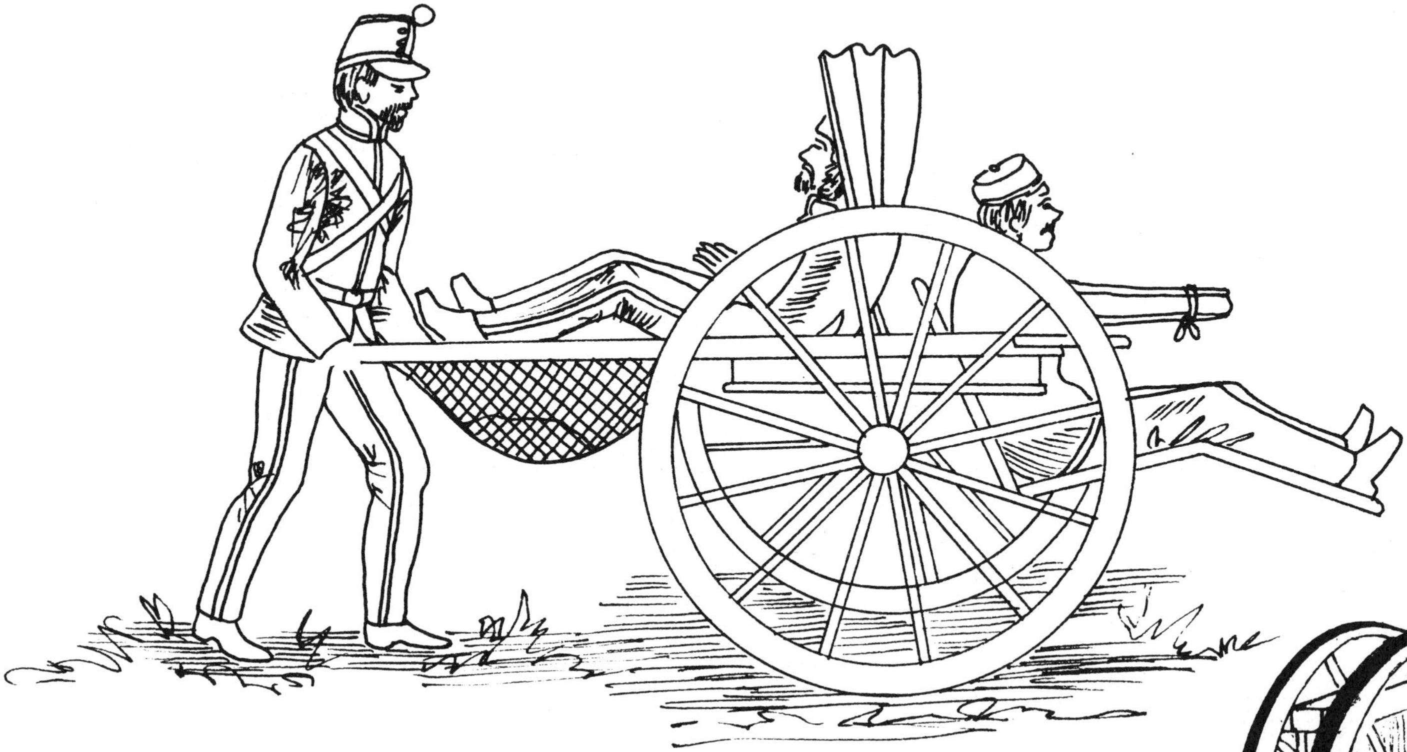

Figure 5-8, Neudorfer's Two-Wheeled Litter for transporting one or two wounded soldiers (European model)

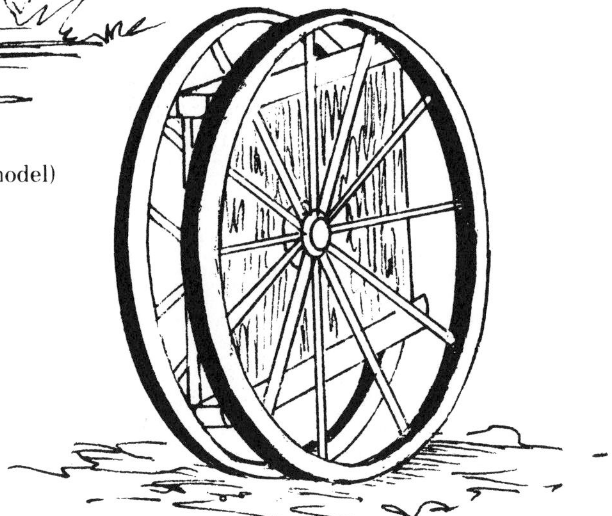

Figure 5-8a, Neudorfer's Litter folded
Redrawn from Longmore's *Treatise, 1866*

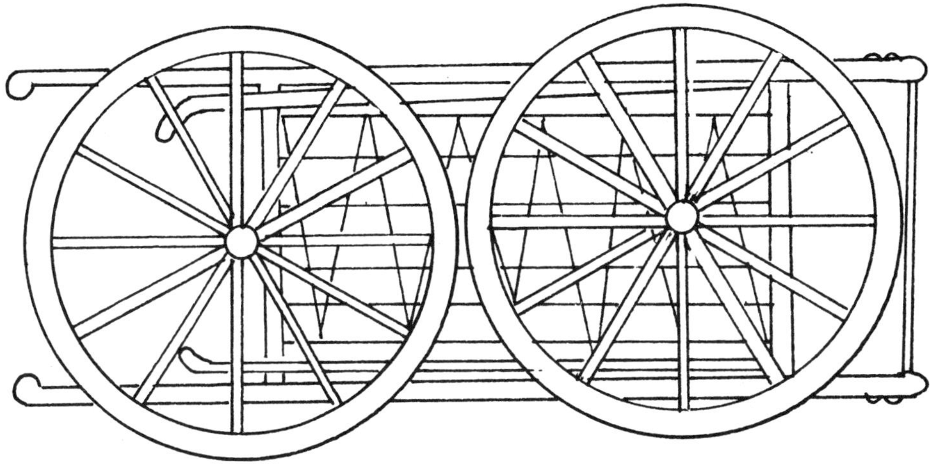

Figure 5-9a, Gablenz's Wheeled Litter arranged for packing
Redrawn from Longmore's *Treatise*, *1866*

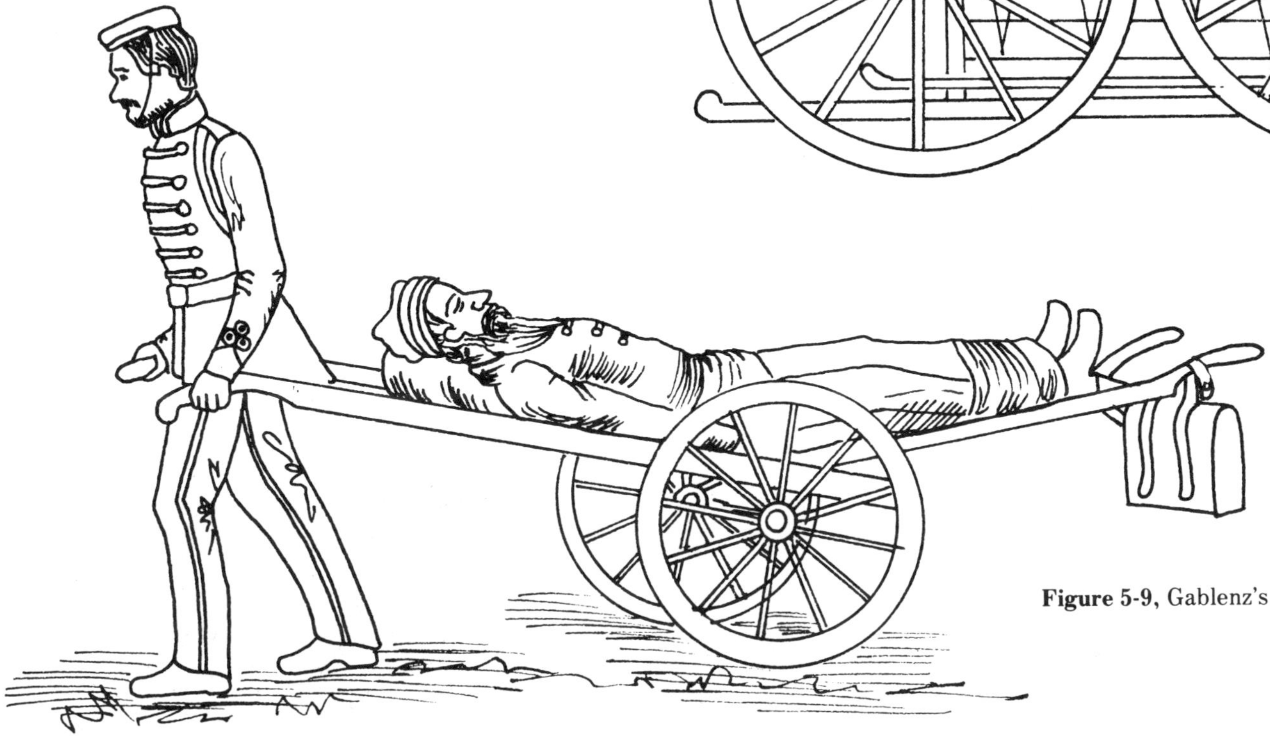

Figure 5-9, Gablenz's Wheeled Litter (European model)

SECTION THREE

Litters Borne by Animals

Two-Horse/Mule Litters

While Army regulations (par. 1298) authorized these litters be furnished to military posts where wheeled vehicles could not travel,[1] records fail to show that any were ever received at the frontier army posts. Furthermore, no evidence has been seen that these were ever used during the Civil War.

Professor Longmore's chief objection to the use of the two-horse litter was that it was uneconomical to use two horses to carry one man.[2] Nevertheless, this type of litter was commonly improvised and used in the western plains. It was easy to construct, tolerably comfortable and was useful in transporting soldiers suffering from amputations, chest, abdomen or hip wounds.

The two-horse litter shown in Figure 2-1 is an ancient form of litter which was often used for carrying important people or for the carriage of sick persons before the introduction of coaches in the sixteenth century. When transporting notable personages, it was fitted with a cab-like structure which afforded some privacy to the individuals riding in the litter.

In America the primary use of the litter was to transport sick and wounded soldiers. Inspector General Randolph B. Marcy of the United States Army, in his "Handbook for Overland Expeditions," gave specific instructions for its construction should a party traveling without ambulance or wagons have one of its members sick or wounded and unable to walk or ride horseback. Marcy's specifications for such a litter were that it be constructed "by taking two poles about twenty feet in length, uniting them by two sticks three feet long lashed across the centre at six feet apart, and stretching a piece of stout canvas, a blanket or hide between them to form a bed." Two gentle horses or mules were then placed between the poles as depicted in the photograph.[3]

The litter authorized by the War Department for issue to the garrisons on the Indian frontier differed but little from the Marcy litter. The regulation army litter, Figure 2-2, consisted of a canvas bed stretched between two poles of ash sixteen feet long and 2-2/3 inches in diameter divided into sections united by strong wrought iron strap hinges. The leading sections were 4-1/2 feet in length, the middle section 8 feet and the rear section 3-1/2 feet in length. The side poles were kept apart by traverses 25 inches in length. The canvas bed was 6 feet by 2 feet 9 inches with the side poles inserted through a wide hem running on each side of the canvas bed. The end sections were furnished with heavy straps and girths. When completed, the litter weighed 88 pounds.[4]

This type of litter was easily constructed on the site of any engagement or skirmish. In addition to its recommended use for westward-bound travelers, it found great favor among the troops fighting in areas devoid of roads. In addition to its use by Surgeon Satterlee during the Seminole War of 1835, reports from other areas substantiate its practicability.

Colonel G.E. Cooper observed its use near Mexico City during one engagement of the Mexican War. Assistant Surgeon Lyman H. Stone used the two-horse litter with good results on an expedition against the Apache Indians in 1852 near Fort Conrad, New Mexico Territory. In the course of the agonizing march of the survivors from the Little Big Horn, June, 1876, many of the wounded were brought to the steamer Far West on two-horse litters constructed under the direction of First Lieutenant Gustavus C. Doane, 2nd U.S. Cavalry. Later that same year, Acting Surgeon Valentine McGillicuddy reported that two-horse litters were used to "semi" advantage in removing casualties after

General Crooks engagement against the Sioux near Slim Buttes, Wyoming Territory. McGillicuddy, as did some other Army Surgeons, favored the travois (which is discussed in a later chapter) over the two-horse litter.

Some of the disadvantages observed by the users of the two-horse litter were that it takes two animals and sometimes two attendants to each animal. The two animals don't always walk in step as it were. One or both animals could stumble thus breaking equipment and throwing the patient to the ground. Animals drafted for this conveyance aren't always gentle nor able to work together. A patient's life may be endangered by animals foundering or stumbling when crossing streams or boggy ground.[5]

Thistle's Single-Horse Litter

In the course of the Florida Campaign against the Indians, Captain H.L. Thistle of the Louisiana Volunteers devised a single-horse litter for the transportation of the wounded through the narrowest of defiles or over the roughest terrain. Before applying for a patent on it in 1837, Captain Thistle offered to furnish fifty complete sets of the litter to the Quartermaster's Department at fifty dollars a set. A complete set included litter, saddle and other necessary appurtenances. A search of the patent office records shows a drawing of the litter as it appears in Figure 2-3, but unfortunately, the specifications are missing.

According to oldtimers at the War Department, the Quartermaster did inspect the litter, but they do not know if the conveyance was ever issued to troops in the field.

Several army officers reporting from the field in 1836 testified favorably on Captain Thistle's single-horse litter as being far superior to the two-horse litter because it could be used as pack saddle when not carrying wounded soldiers. A Major John Mountfort of a U.S. Artillery unit expressed the hope that the War Department would adopt it for the service. But, as we know, they did not. Another favorable testimonial came from a Dr. C.A. Luzenberg who wrote that he "...took pleasure in commending the ingenious saddle constructed by Captain Thistle." Dr. Luzenberg added that he had had ample opportunity to examine various other transports in Europe, and Captain Thistle's was the best of the lot and especially suited to Indian warfare.[6] In addition, the Quartermaster General, Thomas Jesup, after viewing two of the "Thistle Pack Saddles" was of the opinion that they "should prove highly advantageous" and that he had "taken measures to have them fairly tested in the actual service in the field." General Jesup further stated that if the appropriations permitted, he would have them replace other conveyances on hand.[7] However, in spite of the many favorable comments, the records are silent on their use during the Civil War and even on the western frontier.

The Travois

A conveyance that transports sick and wounded in which one end rests on the ground, the other end secured to the animal drawing it. Any reader of Indian or frontier literature has in all probability seen pictures or drawings of this type of litter.

In its simplest form, it consists of two poles, sixteen to seventeen feet long, four to six inches in diameter, with crossbars approximately thirty inches long attached to the two poles to keep them rigid. A piece of canvas, animal hide or other suitable material, is attached to the poles and crosspieces to form a bed for the patient. This type of conveyance can be made on the spot in fifteen minutes or so providing the necessary materials are at hand.

This type of conveyance had been used by the Indians for centuries to transport baggage, children, and sick and ailing relatives.

The early American Colonists resorted to its use on many occasions, and Lewis and Clark called it into service whenever they had to transport sick or injured members of their westward expedition in 1804-1806.

The field service of these primitive conveyances has been proven time and time again. Practically all the military surgeons familiar with their use have praised them for their simple and easy construction, for their ability to move in narrow places, and for the comfort accorded the patients in riding them.

Assistant Surgeon Julius H. Patzki remarked that the military surgeon could always rely on the "old traditional travois" which can ordinarily be constructed on the spot.[1]

On returning from the Powder River Expedition against the Sioux in the winter of 1876, Assistant Surgeon J.R. Gibbon related that the traditional travois with its rude construction and apparent imperfections, was in reality a great boon to the conveyance of casualties. We have already read what Surgeons Munn and Hartsuff had to say about them and we have seen the excellent service the travois rendered after the Little Big Horn.

As it happens with any type of product, someone comes along with an idea for its improvement. The travois was not immune from some tinkering. Several of the military surgeons made efforts to standardize this conveyance. Needless to say, all the proposed models merely added some special appurtenances to the simple Indian model.

For instance, Assistant Surgeon Peter A.J. Cleary proposed that each side pole which forms the shafts be jointed and held in place by an easily removable pin so that the travois could be used as a hand stretcher when that need arose. All dimensions of his travois were comparable to the originals. One feature of interest about Surgeon Cleary's litter, though, was not the litter itself, but the harness. In addition to the regular girth to which the poles were attached, Cleary added a hip strap to pass over the horse's hips and be attached to the shafts of the travois in such a manner that the litter could not be upset should the horse rear up or kick about.

Surgeon Charles Greenleaf proposed a travois similar to Cleary's. The shafts held together by a collar arrangement could be separated when a hand stretcher needed to be used. Nevertheless, none of these proposed models were ever adopted by the U.S. Army. It was content to use the old traditional Indian travois which met the test of time in grand style.

Cacolets (Figure 5-10)

An unusual name for a common conveyance employed by so many European armies in the transportation of their wounded soldiers. The British and French even had cacolets for use on camels.

The term cacolet was thought to have been derived from its resemblance to a container used by the peasants of Bordeaux, France, to carry milk (cacque au lait), however, other authorities point out that there is no basis for that derivation of the term. They say that it actually originated in the Pyrenees Mountains where the word is used to denote a pannier in which supplies and, on occasion, people were carried on mule back. The French found the cacolets of great value in the Algerian campaign and adopted them for general field service.[8]

The cacolet came into prominence in this country during the early years of the Civil War when the already harried officials of the War Department were besieged by citizens clamoring for an official review of their particular cacolet. Fact of the matter is, all of their designs were patterned with a few modifications from designs depicted in Major Delafield's official report on the "Art of War in Europe, 1854-56."

A Mr. W.C.H. Waddell (October, 1861) started the procession of cacolet designers with his proposal to Secretary of War Cameron. No action was taken on Mr. Waddell's proposal. He was followed a month later by Mr. G. Kohler who offered to furnish "mule litters and chairs" (cacolets) patterned, with few slight modifications, from those used in the Crimean War. The War Department apparently found merit in Mr. Kohler's conveyance and ordered 300 of them be purchased at $70.00 per set, $21,000 in all.[9]

Lawrence, Bradley and Pardee of New Haven, Connecticut, applied for a patent on their cacolet (1861), but the U.S. Patent Index does not show that a patent was issued for this litter. It did have serious disadvantages, though, as it was a heavy 131 pounds, the chair could not be detached from the saddle, and the whole apparatus was structurally weak and inconvenient.

The War Department was kept busy convening Medical Boards of Officers to examine all of these contraptions. Finally, in September, 1862, after disapproving a cacolet designed by Mr. Slade Davis, they recommended that no further cacolets be purchased from any source whatever.

But whether the War Department accepted this Board's recommendation or not, it didn't stop the eager litter and cacolet designers from beating a path to its door. Mr. Davis was followed by a Mr. J. Jones of New York City. His litter varied from the others in that it could be removed from its saddle and used as hand stretchers or hospital beds. Next came another gentleman from New York City, Mr. E.P. Woodcock, whose proposed litter included an outlandish outrigger contrivance extending along the saddle from pommel to cantle. It was exhibited at the Paris Exposition in 1867, but received as cold a reception there as at home. Mr. Woodcock was followed in early fall of 1863 by the Spencer and Nichols Company representatives who

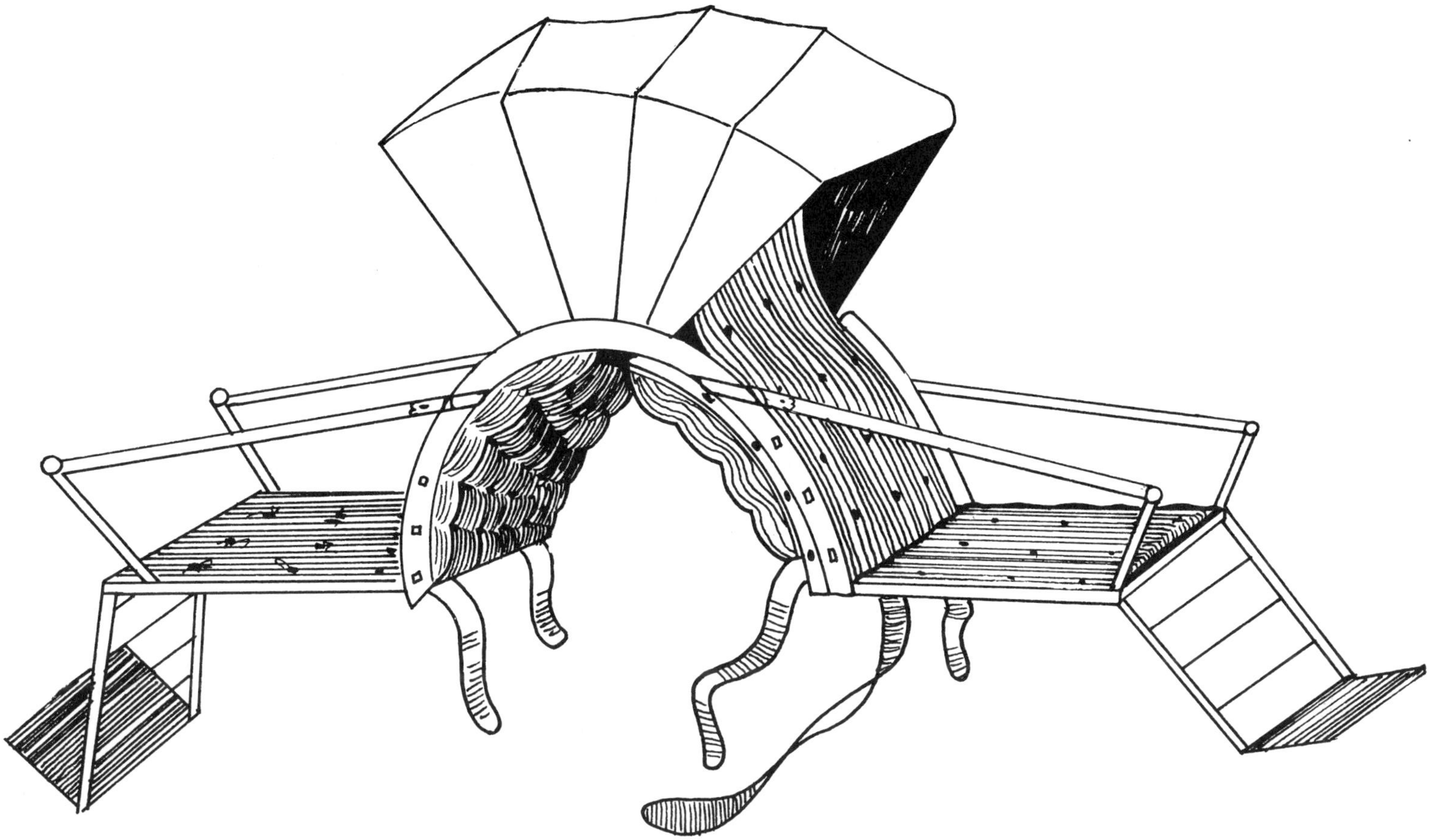

Figure 5-10, Cacolet by Lawrence, Bradley and Pardee (Kohler's exception seats faced forward, no canopy)
Redrawn from *Medical-Surgical History, War of Rebellion,* Part III, Vol. II

submitted an "adjustable ambulance pack saddle." Lightness, simplicity, strength, efficiency, adjustability, and cheapness were its chief merits. The Board mildly agreed, but turned the design down. Spencer and Nichols had scarcely left the War Offices before another supplicant with proposals in hand came up the steps of the War Office. They wasted their time; their pattern was rejected by a weary Board of ambulance examiners.[10]

Medical Director of the Army of the Potomac, Charles S. Tripler, as well as his successor, Major Jonathan Letterman, early in the war urged the adoption of horse litters for military units serving in regions impractical for wheeled ambulances. Twelve of these were sent to the Army in the Shenandoah Valley. Another supply of cacolets and litters was issued to the Army of the Potomac for its advance on Richmond in May, 1862. Just before the Battle of Fair Oaks (May 31-June 1, 1862), Surgeon Frank H. Hamilton reported that his Fourth Corps had received eight cacolets and litters. They were used the first day of the battle, but the horses carrying them were so impatient and restless that six of the cacolets were broken. Surgeon Hamilton further observed that mules were better for this purpose than horses though they, too, had to be trained for this duty.[11] This is the only incident wherein cacolets were ever reportedly used in actual battle conditions in this country.

The Quartermaster had an ample supply of cacolets on hand—remember the government had purchased 300 of the Kohler pattern. One of the persistent problems plaguing the Quartermaster Department and the military surgeon in the field was the dearth of trained mules or horses to carry the cacolets. At one point early in the war, the Surgeon General Hammond requested that 100 cacolets be sent to the Army of the Potomac after Antietam, but the animals selected to bear these litters were so unruly that the litters couldn't be used.

At another time, General Hammond made another requisition for 150 mules with drivers. He proposed to have them drilled with cacolets before being put into service, but this attempt, like all the others, failed as a result of which this type of conveyance piled up in the Quartermaster's warehouses. The Quartermaster General became so concerned at the high cost of the expenses connected with this equipment that, unless ordered by higher authority, he would not expend another cent of public funds for its continuance.

The failure of this type of ambulance conveyance in our armies seems due more to lack of acceptance on the part of the military commanders than to any defects in the litters themselves, even though they appeared rather cumbersome. With trained animals and efficient personnel, they probably could have been successful. Yet, Surgeon George V. Suckely, in a letter to Surgeon John H. Brinton (March 30, 1863) declared that there were no cacolets in his corps, and he didn't want any. They are "only troublesome and barberous encumberances cruel alike to the wounded and to the pack animals."[12]

Although the Civil War had ended and the defenders of the Union and the Confederacy had gone home, there were still certain inventors about the land beating a path to the War Department's office in Washington. They were all imbued with the desire of, and the hope that, the military authorities would adopt their ideas as being the most efficient in transporting the wounded soldiers.

Rooker's Saddle Attachment

One such fellow who assailed the busy offices of the War Department was Mr. W.B. Rooker of Prince George's County, Maryland. He had under his arm drawings for a saddle attachment that could easily be used by any slightly wounded cavalryman.

Rooker's creation was so made that it could be fitted to the regula-

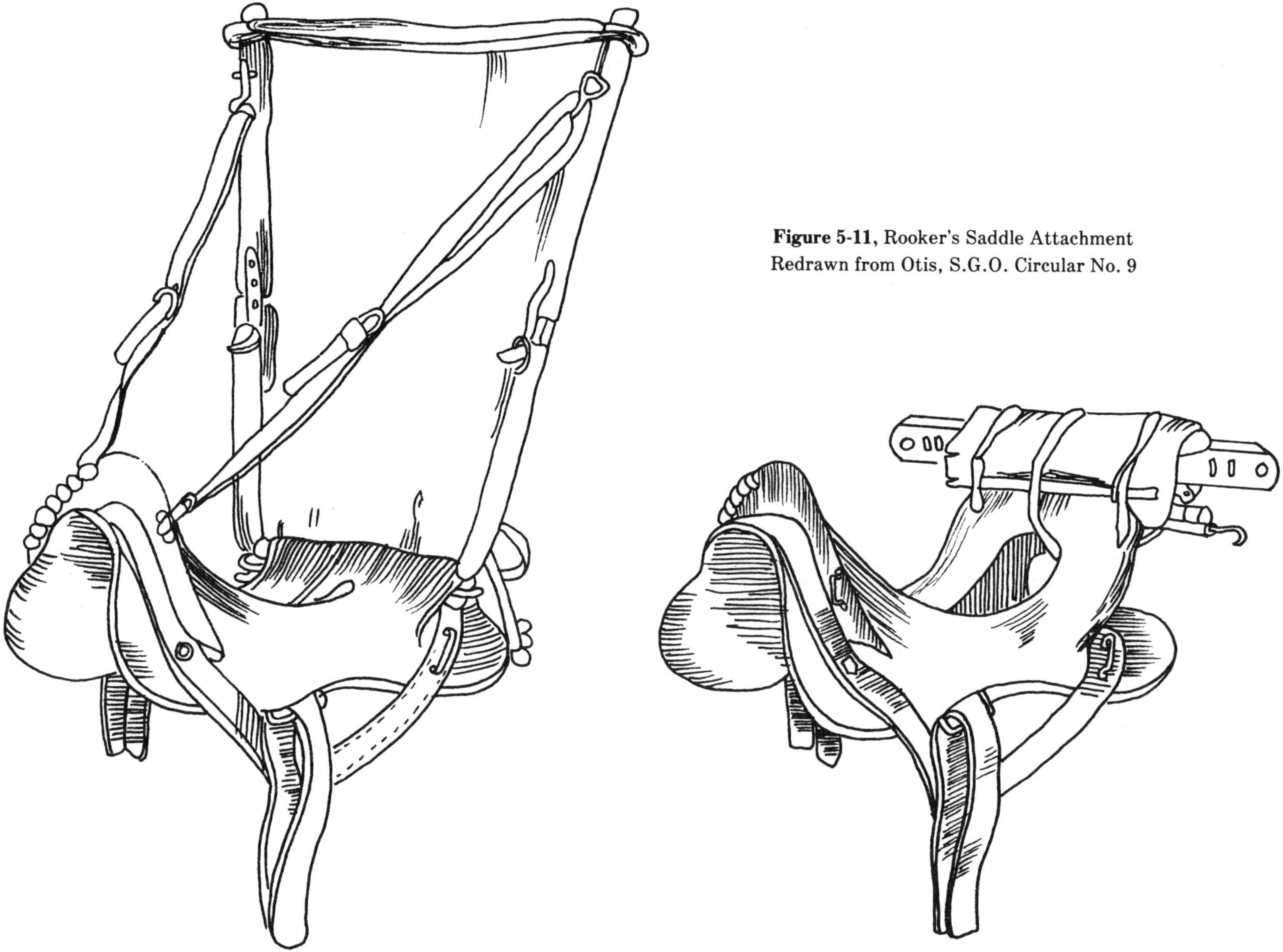

Figure 5-11, Rooker's Saddle Attachment
Redrawn from Otis, S.G.O. Circular No. 9

tion cavalry saddle. It consisted of two upright bars hinged in the middle. A crossbar was attached to these two bars which supported a piece of canvas used as a back rest. Two leather straps with buckles were so arranged that they could be taken in or let out, thus adjusting the back of the attachment to suit the rider's condition. When not in use, the canvas back could be rolled down in a compact bundle. The weight of the contraption was a mere 4-3/8 pounds. It could be operational in five minutes.

Rooker's proposal met with little official favor, but the man was so insistent that several of his contraptions were ordered made up at the Watervliet Arsenal, New York. The Board of Medical Officers, which was convened in early 1875 to examine and report on the Rooker Saddle Attachment, didn't think it wise to burden the already overburdened cavalryman with this piece of useless equipment. Nevertheless, the Board ordered that it be given a field trial.

The War Department then sent a few of these contrivances to the Rock Island Arsenal in April, 1875—three were sent to General George A. Custer's command in Dakota Territory, two to Fort Laramie, three to Fort Leavenworth, and one each to Fort Brown, W.T., and Colonel Grierson's command. Soon reports on the value of this attachment began to filter into the War Department in Washington. All the reports were adverse. "I have examined and tested the new ambulance saddle, and for practical use, consider it inferior to many, if not all the packs and litters commonly constructed..." so reported Captain J. Mix, 2d. U.S. Cavalry, Fort Brown, W.T. Other comments were in the same vein. However, it was left to General William T. Sherman to dismiss the entire experiment once and for all. He unequivocally declared "...I have examined the Rooker ambulance saddle and do not hesitate to pronounce it useless in war and peace..."[13]

Before ringing down the curtain on litters borne by animals, it will

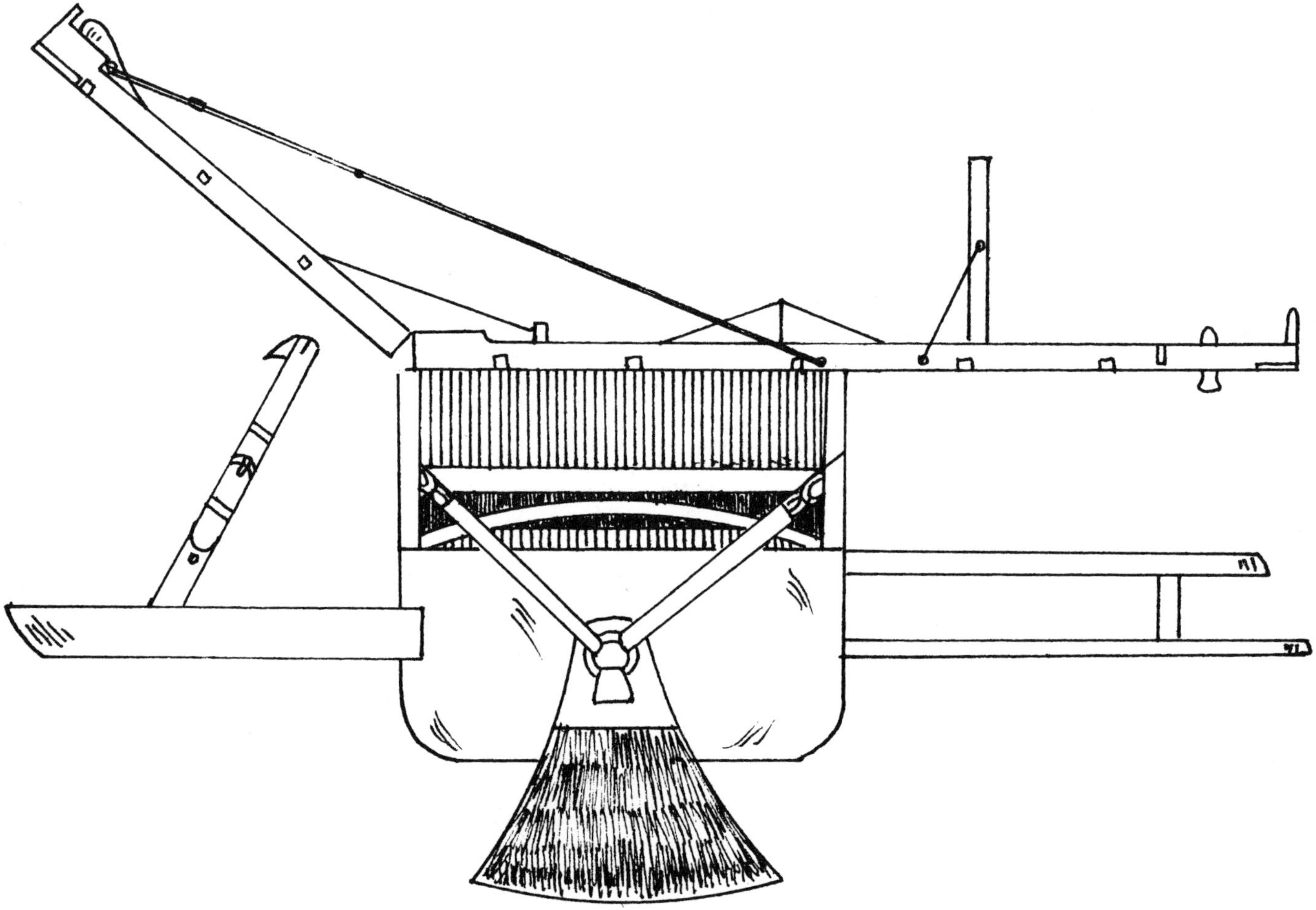

Figure 5-12a, McElderry's Single-Mule Litter (side view)

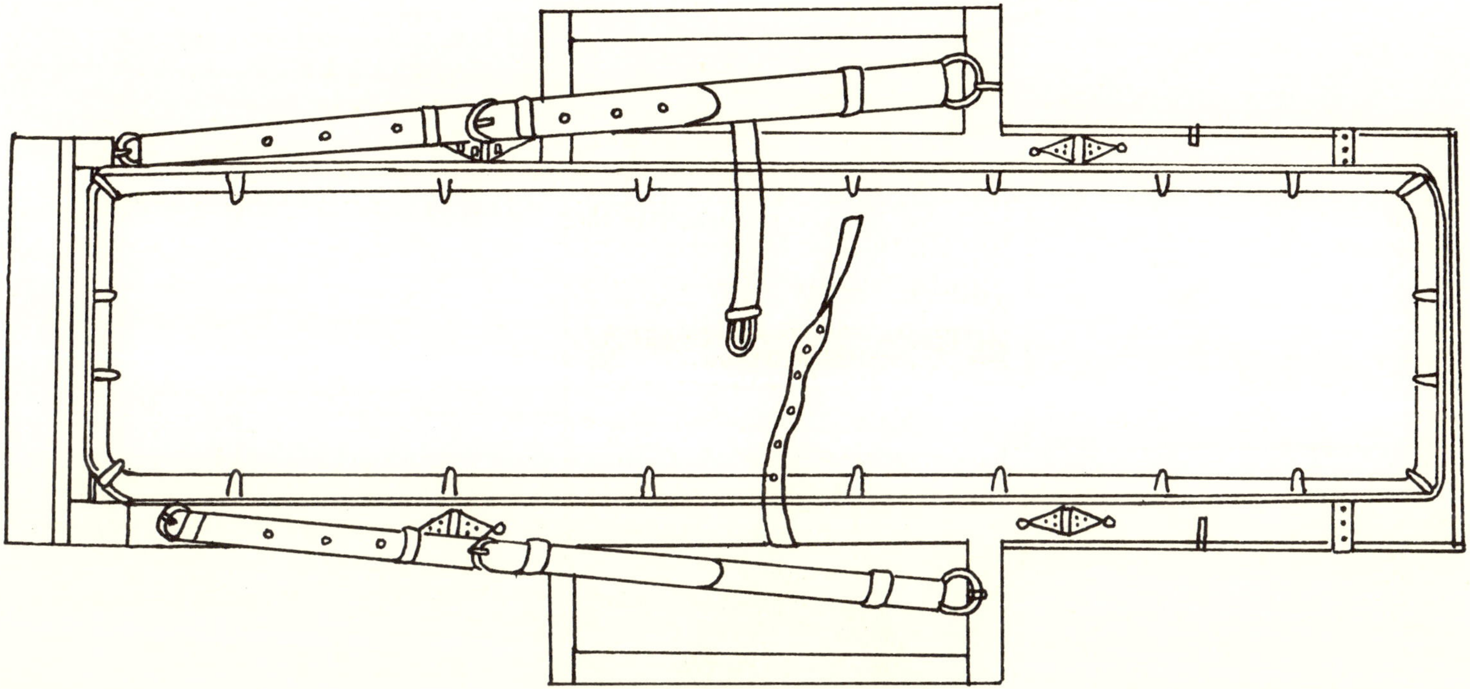

Figure 5-12b, McElderry's Single-Mule Litter (top view)
Redrawn from Otis, S.G.O. Circular No. 9

be well to look at one more. This one was designed by Surgeon Henry McElderry, a veteran of many western Indian campaigns. Like Captain Thistle's single-horse litter, the width of McElderry's litter did not exceed the flanks of the animal bearing it. This narrow width allowed the mule or horse to pass through narrow defiles, canyons or roads without incidence.

Surgeon McElderry's litter boasted several advantages: (1) Litter could be folded completely to accommodate a load of forage or supplies on its return trip to the combat zone. (2) On return from the combat zone, the litter could be unfolded and made ready to carry a wounded soldier to the hospital area. (3) By use of adjustable iron supports, the litter could be adjusted to any desired position. (4) It would be attached to the Mexican aparejo which was universally used in most army pack trains. (5) Litter is well balanced and thus comfortable to the pack animal and the patient. (6) A canvas canopy could be provided, if necessary. (7) The heavy canvas bed opens at one end so that straw or hay can be stuffed into the bed. (8) The combined weight of the litter and aparejo is but 104 pounds. Although no records of costs were found, a fair estimate would be sixty to seventy dollars.

The Quartermaster's Department issued 700-800 of these to the troops, but with the exception of its use during the Modoc Campaign of 1872-73, it was little used and set aside. It was easier for the frontier regulars to make a travois or a two-horse litter on the spot than to carry ready-made ones in the ambulance trains.[14]

SECTION FOUR
Ambulance Wagons

Wagons specifically designed and constructed for the transportation of the army's wounded did not appear on the battle fronts of this country until after the publication of Major Delafield's prestigious report, "The Art of War in Europe, 1854-56." Coincidentally with the publication of this report, Doctor Israel Moses, formerly Army Assistant Surgeon, 1847-55, now private physician of New York City, proposed a unique type of ambulance wagon. Whether Doctor Moses had read Delafield's description of European ambulance wagons is not known, but a few months later, a Board of Medical Officers consisting of Surgeons Richard S. Satterlee, C.H. Laub and Assistant Surgeon C.H. Crane convened (March 2, 1858) in Washington to examine the Moses creation.

The Moses (Figure 5-13)

1. Seating for eighteen persons, fourteen inside and four on the front seat with the driver.
2. Seats could be arranged to accommodate one to three men lying down, and if necessary, one or two more patients could be carried on a piece of canvas suspended from the inside of the ambulance top.
3. Attached to either side of the top of the wagon was a tent-like arrangement which could be let down to form a temporary hospital tent. When not in use, it could be rolled up along the top edges of the ambulance. This portable hospital tent obviated the necessity of carrying extra personnel to set up hospital tents.
4. The wagon was entered from the rear by two steps.
5. Body of ambulance: 13'8" long, 4'4" wide, height ground to top, 8'4", inside head room, 5'.

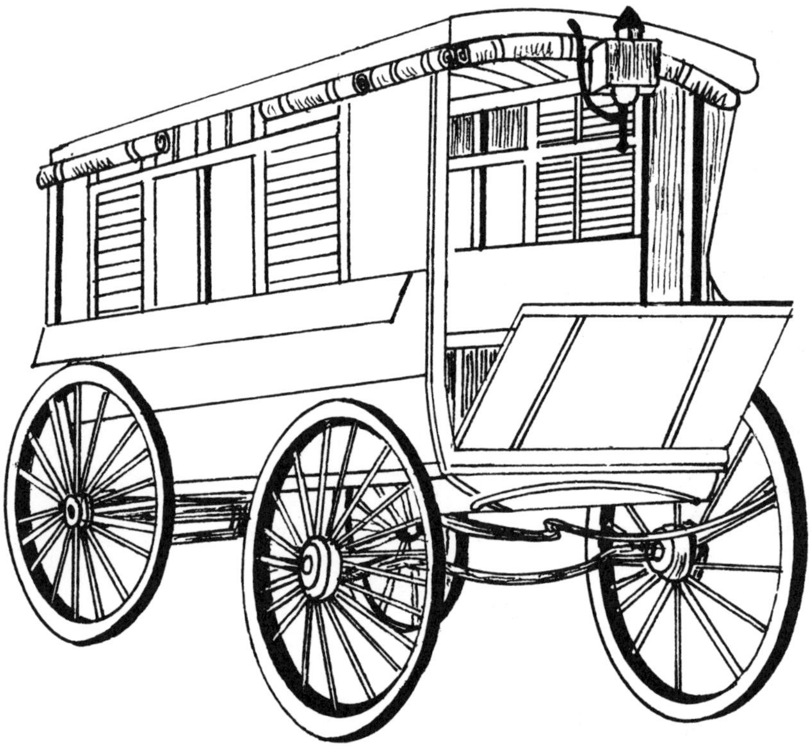

Figure 5-13, The Moses Ambulance Wagon (oblique view)

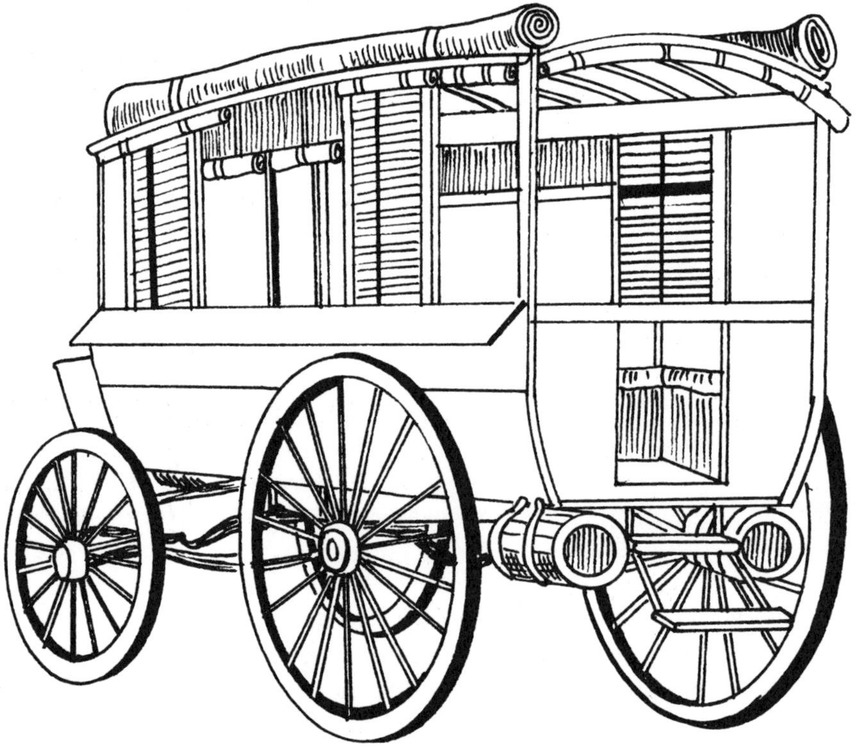

Figure 5-13a, The Moses Ambulance Wagon (rear view)

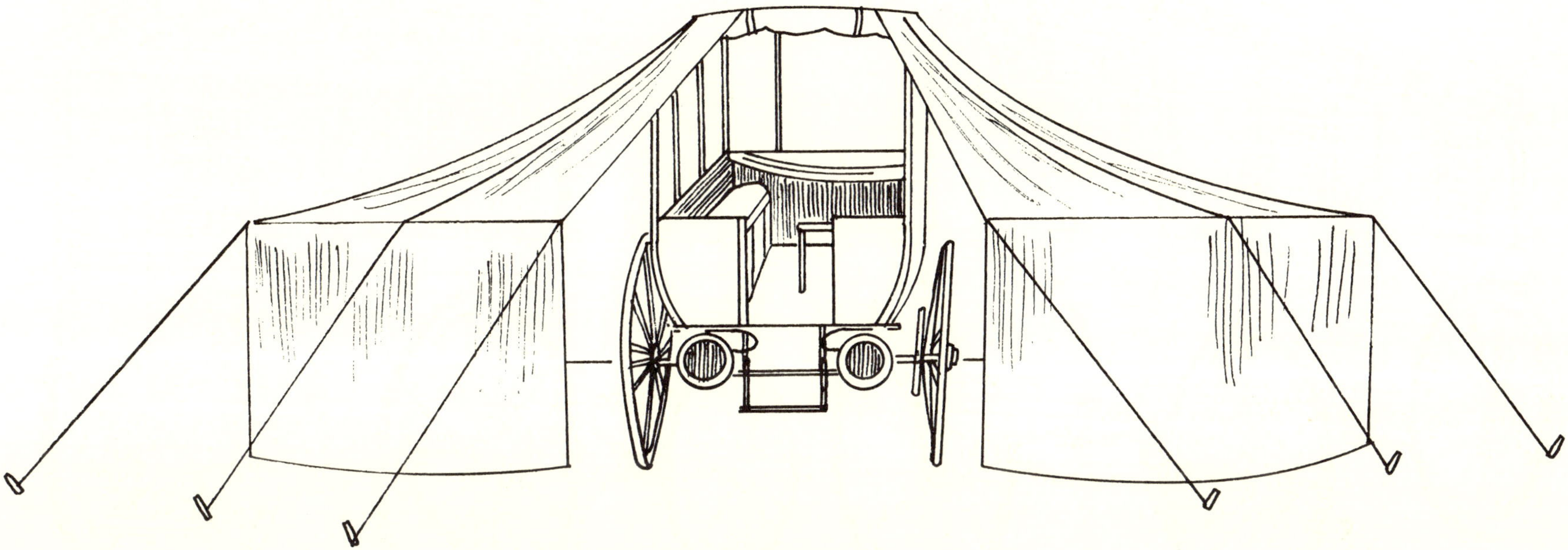

Figure 5-13b, The Moses Ambulance Wagon and Tent
Redrawn from *Medical-Surgical History, War of Rebellion,* Part III, Vol. II

6. Weight, empty: 2,115 pounds. Required six horses to draw it.
7. Equipment: Two five-gallon kegs carried in built-in receptacles rear of wagon. Chests for necessary medical and surgical supplies. Removable door for use as writing desk, amputation table, or for dispensing medicines. The regulation ambulance lantern, carried by all ambulances, could be moved to the rear, if desired.

Comments- The Board thought that this ambulance, although rather heavy, was well adapted to field service, that it was comfortable for patients, and that the hospital tent provided valuable and useful shelter for the wounded. No official action seems to have followed the Board's recommendation, hence, none of these ambulances were ever built.[1]

"No man who has ever ridden in the two-wheeled ambulance would willingly get into one again, even if well." The Tommy Yanks who observed or possibly had the misfortune to ride in one of these two-wheelers nicknamed it "Avalanche" because when it was driven, it so often violently ejected its patients to the ground. These two-wheelers were well suited for hauling provisions or to serve as pleasure vehicles, but as ambulance wagons, they were useless. Why then did the Union Army use so many during the first years of the war?

It all started in October, 1859, when a Board of Medical Officers to examine ambulances, consisting of Surgeons Clement A. Finley, R.S. Satterlee, C.S. Tripler, J.M. Cuyler, and Assistant Surgeon R.H. Coolidge, recommended that ambulance transportation ought to be furnished for forty men per thousand, and that both the two-wheeled and four-wheeled ambulance wagons are necessary. Furthermore, the Board opined that a two-wheeled ambulance wagon was the *best* for conveyance of the dangerously sick or wounded men. The Board hesitated to favor one over the other (possibly because both Surgeons

Finley and Coolidge sat on the Board), therefore, it recommended that both two-wheelers be built and issued to the army.

The Finley (Figure 5-14)

Sills	- 7'6" long out to out.
Body	- 6'9" long out to out, 4'1¼" wide, 4'4½" high.
Side Panels	- 18" high, ½" thick; 4 posts 1¼" x 1".
Tail Board	- Let down type, same height as side panels.
Seats	- 21" wide, bar behind top of each seat. Cushion 13"; seats hinged to raise in center.
Frame	- White ash; side panels of poplar.
Shafts	- White hickory, 11'3" long. Singletree fastened by clevis and bolt. Prop stick 2'6½" connected to the shaft.
Springs	- All half springs, front spring 3'8" long, 2" wide, 7 plates (leaves); back spring, 3'8" long, 2" wide, 6 plates. Side springs, 4'5" long, 2" wide, 6 plates.
Litter	- Frame 6'4¾" long, 22" wide, sides 6" wide, ½" thick. Legs of litter also form the handles. Four small trunk rollers set in each corner of frame so that the litter can be rolled in or out.
Mattress	- Best ticking with curled hair; pillows stuffed with hair.
Wheels	- 4'7" high, hubs 7" x 9". Tires secured to wheels by bolts. Wheels secured to axles by a newly patented washer and linchpin.
Markings	- Each side of ambulance to be marked U.S. All other parts lettered U.S.
Equipment	- Head lining oil cloth, heavy oil cloth curtains on each side, one glass in center of curtain.

Two hooks inside ambulance to hold rifles or muskets.

Baggage crate slung under bottom of floor. Water keg 14" x 10" hooked into the tail piece of the sills.

Special - As in all government contracts for ambulance wagons, a special provision was included which read: "It is agreed and distinctly understood that the several parts of any one ambulance will agree and exactly fit those of any other so as to require no numbering or arranging for putting together..."[2]

The Coolidge

Built at the same time as the FINLEY, was quite similar with these exceptions: The body, 7' long, 4' wide was set on platform springs. When reference to two-wheeled ambulances was made by name, the COOLIDGE never seemed to show up.

The War Department ordered 200 of the Finley's be constructed. Several firms built these ambulance wagons. Joseph Crowell of Rahway, New Jersey (June 22, 1861) contracted to build fifty at $150.00 each. Charles Elliott of New York City built fifty at the same price as did G.D. Cook & Co. of New Haven, Connecticut.[3]

That these two-wheelers were unsafe, flimsy, and often "shook to pieces" is amply borne out by reports from the field. Surgeon C.E. Boyle, Ninth Regiment, Ohio Volunteers, reporting from the Shenandoah Valley, stated that they were entirely unfit for use and that after a march of fifty miles or so, they fell apart.[4]

Surgeon Tripler, Medical Director of the Army of the Potomac in a letter to Acting Surgeon General Wood (April 25, 1862), bears out Surgeon Boyle's comment by stating that from his observation and concurrent testimony of all concerned he found the two-wheelers to be

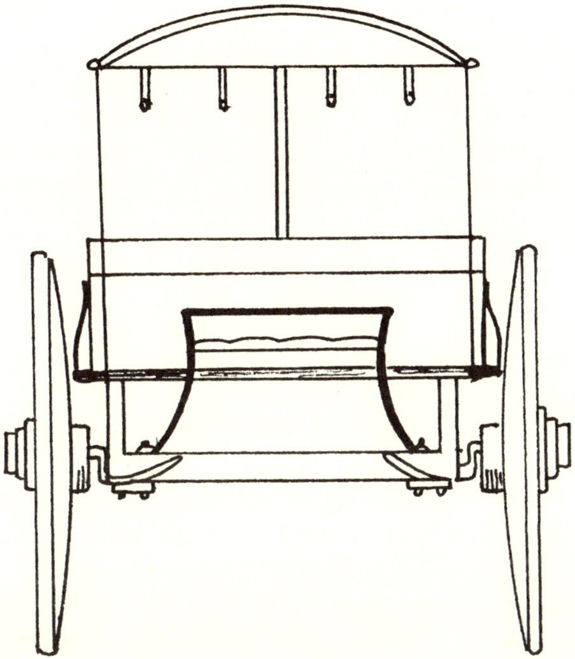

Figure 5-14, The Finley Two-Wheeled Ambulance (front view)

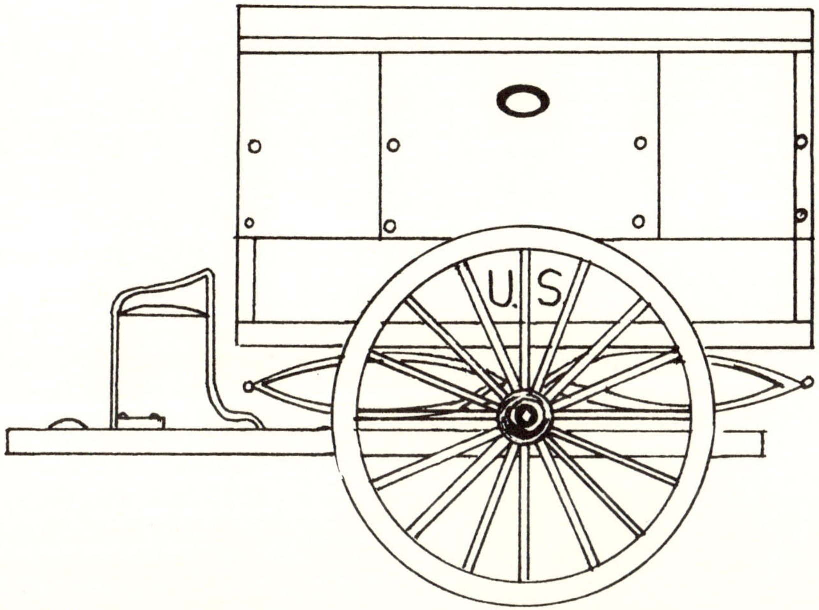

Figure 5-14a, The Finley Two-Wheeled Ambulance (side view)
Redrawn from *Medical-Surgical History, War of Rebellion,* Part III, Vol. II

totally unfit. "Their motion is unbearable and excruciating, men beg to be taken out of them, and wounded officers have insisted on leaving them, in one case, mounting a horse, in another taking a seat in front of a four-wheeled ambulance." Tripler closed his letter with these words, "Hope no more be built."[5] Happily for all concerned, no more "Avalanches" were built after 1862. They were supplanted by the four-wheeled vehicles of which the Tripler was the first.

Named for Surgeon Charles S. Tripler, a member of the 1859 Board which approved the two-wheelers. Available records do not show whether Tripler had a hand in designing this ambulance or not. This ambulance wagon did prove most serviceable in the first years of the war. It was constructed to carry ten men, four lying at length and six seated. It required four horses to pull it.

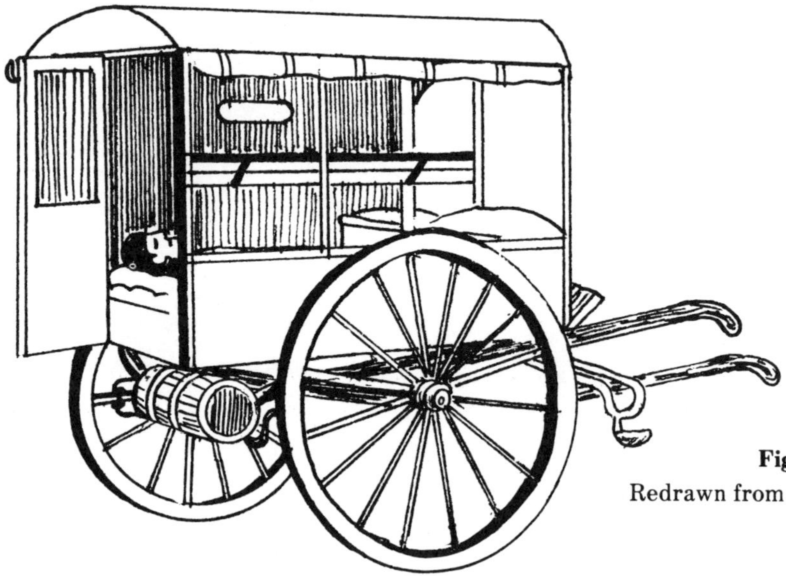

Figure 5-14b, The Coolidge Two-Wheeled Ambulance
Redrawn from *Medical & Surgical History, War of Rebellion,* Part III, Vol. II

The Tripler (Figure 5-15)

Sills	- 11' long out to out (including foot board), 8 studs on each side. Sides are solid panels 30" high.
Body	- 8'9½" long from tail piece to box in front, 4' wide in the clear, 5' high in center from floor to ridge-pole. The top is oval, 6 bows 2" x 5/8" fastened to rails and studs with screws.
Top	- Heavy canvas cover #2 duck. Three curtains on each side, and a front and back curtain.
Springs	- Back spring is 4'2" long from center to center; side springs back 3'10" x 2¾" wide with 6 plates; side springs front 3'10" long, 2¾" wide, 6 plates.
Axles	- 1¾" square, nuts on ends; boxes 8½" long.
Wheels	- Back wheels 4'8" high without tires; hubs 7½" x 10". Tire 2" wide. Front wheels 3'8" high without tire; hubs 7¼" x 10".
Houns or Hounds	- Half houns 2' long, 5th wheel 2' diameter. Whole houns 4'4" long.
Double Tires	- 4' long.
Tongue	- 10'6" long; a hook with an eye in it on top of tongue to attach lead bar for lead horses.
Litter	- 6'7½" long, 32" wide. Solid bottom, mattress of heavy oil cloth stuffed with curled hair. The litters are designed so that they can be easily handled. There are 4 litters for each wagon, 4 small pillows and 2 cushions, one for driver and one for back seat. The upper tier of litters same as lower. A hook fastened to the floor keeps litters in place when vehicle is moving.

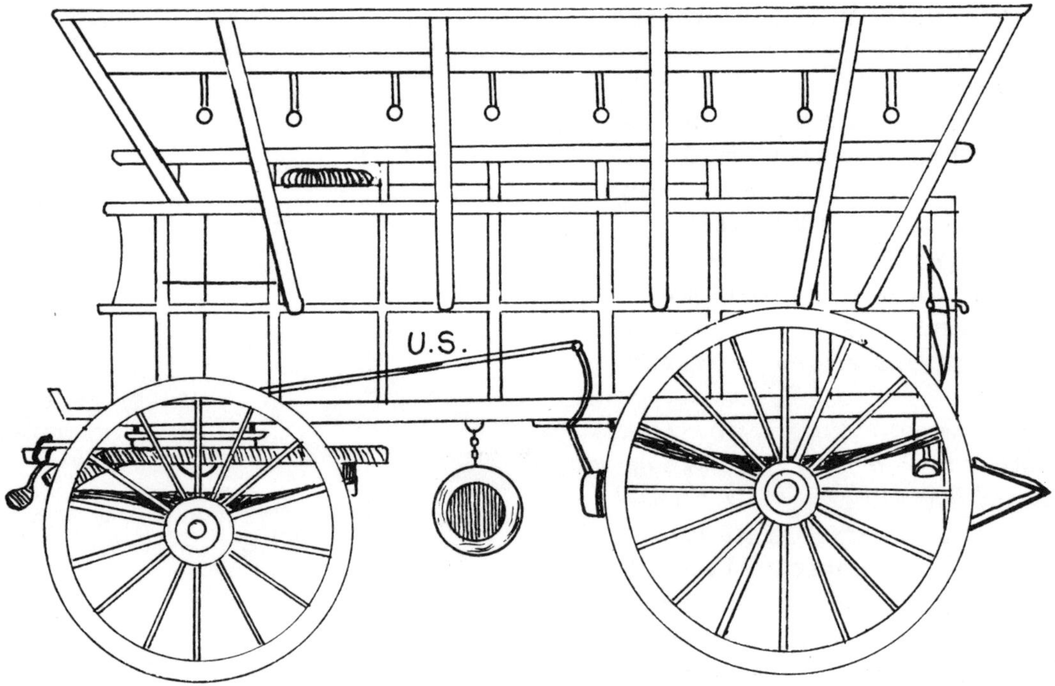

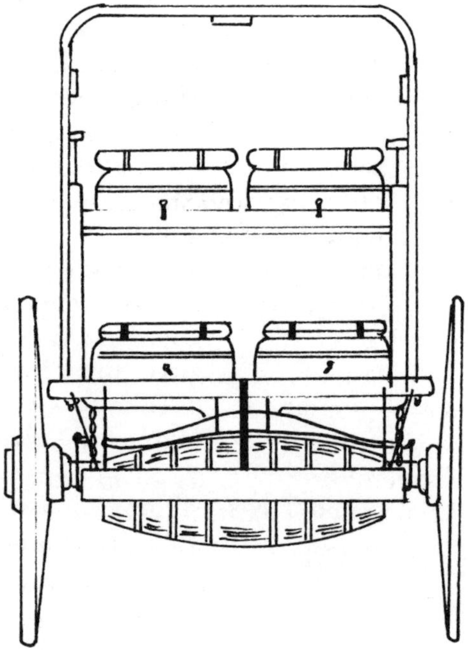

Figure 5-15, The Tripler Ambulance Wagon (side view)

Figure 5-15a, The Tripler Ambulance Wagon (rear view)

Redrawn from *Medical-Surgical History, War of Rebellion,* Part III, Vol. II

Equipment - Water keg 3'8" long. Thirteen inch center tapering to 10" at ends. Hung from the sills by chain and hooks. A box 18" wide, 11½" long for carrying medical supplies form the driver's seat.

Markings - Each side of ambulance marked with U.S. All other parts lettered U.S.[6]

The interior of the ambulance wagon was so fitted out that it could be removed, making it available for the transportation of medical supplies. This ambulance wagon was fairly heavy and required four horses to pull it. Captain Van Vliet of Fort Leavenworth, K.T. (July 28, 1860) remarked that the Tripler "runs heavy if not heavier than six mule baggage wagons."[7]

While the Tripler was used throughout the war, construction of new ones ceased in 1862. Figures for the total number of Triplers purchased and issued is difficult to find as many records concerning ambulances refer to them as "four-wheeled ambulances" and not by name. An educated guess would be that several hundred were issued to the military units. Cost of this ambulance ranged from a low of $147 (December, 1861, built by M.W. Woods of Philadelphia) to a high of $275 for those built by Benjamin Stevens of Cincinnati (June, 1861).[8]

Seats - Two cushioned benches were attached to the sides of the interior running the full length of the body. Seats fastened to the benches by hinges could be raised to form beds for patients. The seating arrangement could easily be altered to carry four patients lying down.

Weight - 700-800 pounds.

Springs - Four Elliptical springs 3'3" x 2"; 6 plates. Two of the springs placed transversely, front and back, other two front and back, side springs.

Wheels	- Hind wheels white oak or hickory thoroughly seasoned, 4'1" high; hubs 8" x 6¾"; 16 spokes in wheel felloes in 2 pieces. Front wheels same material as hind wheels. Tires best refined iron 1¼" x 3/8". Eight bolts to fasten each tire on wheel.
Running Gear	- To be made of the best quality of seasoned white oak or hickory.
Painting	- Two coats of lead-color and 3 coats of bronze-color paint on body and running gear; striped with green paint; 1 coat of varnish on body and running gear.
Markings	- Each side of body marked U.S. All parts lettered U.S.
Equipment	- Water keg 18" long; 9½" center tapered to 8½" on each end. To be carried in back panel of the body. Box 11½" x 12½" with lid and hinges for carrying medical supplies.
Special Provisions	- This contract, as did all others pertaining to ambulances, stipulated that the ambulance would be so constructed that any parts could be interchanged with any other ambulance of this same type.[9]

The costs of this ambulance varied from a low of $119 during the first years of the war to a high of $305 toward the end of the conflict. For example, Henry Simons of Philadelphia (July 24, 1862) agreed to build 100 of the Wheelings for $119 each. By fall, the costs had risen to $145. During 1864, the Quartermaster General had to pay $235 each for the ambulances. And, probably because of storage of materials and wartime inflation, several Philadelphia firms raised the cost to an astronomical $305.[10] After the war, the cost settled back to a fairly steady figure of $227-235 for a Wheeling.[11]

The Wheeling continued to be built well into the later years of the war. The only complaint found against the Wheeling was made by Surgeon General John K. Barnes to the Secretary of War (March 31, 1876). The General stated that the ambulance could not be easily turned out of narrow roads to make way for artillery trains or bodies of marching troops. Hence, in the Civil War, it was necessary to keep hospital trains at a greater distance from the actual field of battle than desirable.[12] Incidentally, General Barnes was one of the very few military men who had any praise for the Finley two-wheelers.

Many of those rugged, well-constructed Wheelings followed the military units west to become an important link in the transportation of wounded frontier regulars.

Toward the closing years of the Great Conflict, a still better ambulance wagon than the popular, rugged Wheeling appeared on the scene. It was an ambulance wagon constructed on a design furnished by Brigadier General Daniel H. Rucker of the Quartermaster's Department, and built at the government shops in Washington.

All of these light, four-wheeled ambulance wagons were quite similar in design, materials and construction. The most noticeable difference was in the kind of springs used, elliptical or platform. As far as accommodation of patients was concerned, both the Rucker and Wheeling carried the same.

The Rucker (Figure 5-18)

Sills	- 9'7" including footboard.
Body	- Eight feet six inches long; 4'2" wide out to out; botton 1/2" planed pine boards. Seven studs on side of body, 4 bows mortised to sills of body. Headroom inside 4'10". Tailgate whole width of the body.

Litters	- On the floor were two stretchers suitable for carrying one patient each. Stretchers had usual handles; ran on elastic rollers for ease in loading and unloading. Stretchers were so hinged that they could be used as seats. If necessary to carry more patients in a recumbent position four stretchers, could be slung from the top of the ambulance. Stretcher space is ventilated by four lattice openings on each side of the body panels.
Springs	- The body rests on four platform springs. The 4 side springs are 3'7" x 1½", 7 plates. Cross springs are 4' x 1½", 7 plates. Connected to body by couplers and hangers, side springs set on wooden blocks, clipped to axles.
Running Gear	- Best seasoned hickory.
Wheels	- Back wheels hickory, 4'2" high; front wheels hickory, 3'6" high. Hubs of best gum 6½" x 9" with iron bands on each end. Tires 1½" wide, 3/8" thick, fastened to wheel by 8 bolts.
Covering	- Top of body 12 ounce cotton duck, 3 roll-up curtains on each side of same material, as also the back curtain.
Equipment	- Box for medical supplies. Water keg 16" long, 9" center, tapering to 7" each end. Water kegs carried in space provided in body of ambulance.
Weight	- 1,120 pounds. Exceeds the Wheeling by several hundred pounds, but it is a larger wagon.[13]

Cost of the Rucker manufactured by same firms that built the other ambulances averaged between $225-$250 each.

This ambulance won prizes at the Paris Exposition, 1867, where many ambulances and litters of European and American design were shown. Its rugged construction and ease in handling soon made it a favorite of the frontier military even when replaced by the 1878 "Red Cross" pattern.

As it must happen to all kinds of equipment, it wears out, is destroyed, broken or missing. All of these troubles happened to the ambulances. Parts of these ambulances were, of course, manufactured by some of the same firms that built ambulances and wagons. A quick review of some representative items and prices taken at random from contracts made by the Quartermaster's Department should prove interesting.

Prices for Years 1863-1867

Buttons for ambulance curtains	\$.14 per gross
Faucets for ambulance water kegs	\$.12-\$.13 each
Door handles with locks	\$.50 each
Hames for harness	\$.86 each
Water kegs	\$1.07-\$1.50 each
Four-horse whips	\$.72 each
Two-horse whips	\$.59-\$.63 each
Ambulance bows	\$1.50 per set of 4
Two-horse harness	\$43.96 each
Snaffle bits	\$.20 each
Axle boxes 7½" x 1½"; 8½" x 1½"	\$.30-\$.60 each
Wheel spokes, front	\$.05½-\$.10 each
Wheel spokes, back	\$.05½-\$.07 each
Hubs	\$.50 each
Springs	\$.24½ per lb.
Felloes	\$2.85-\$3.50 set of 2[14]

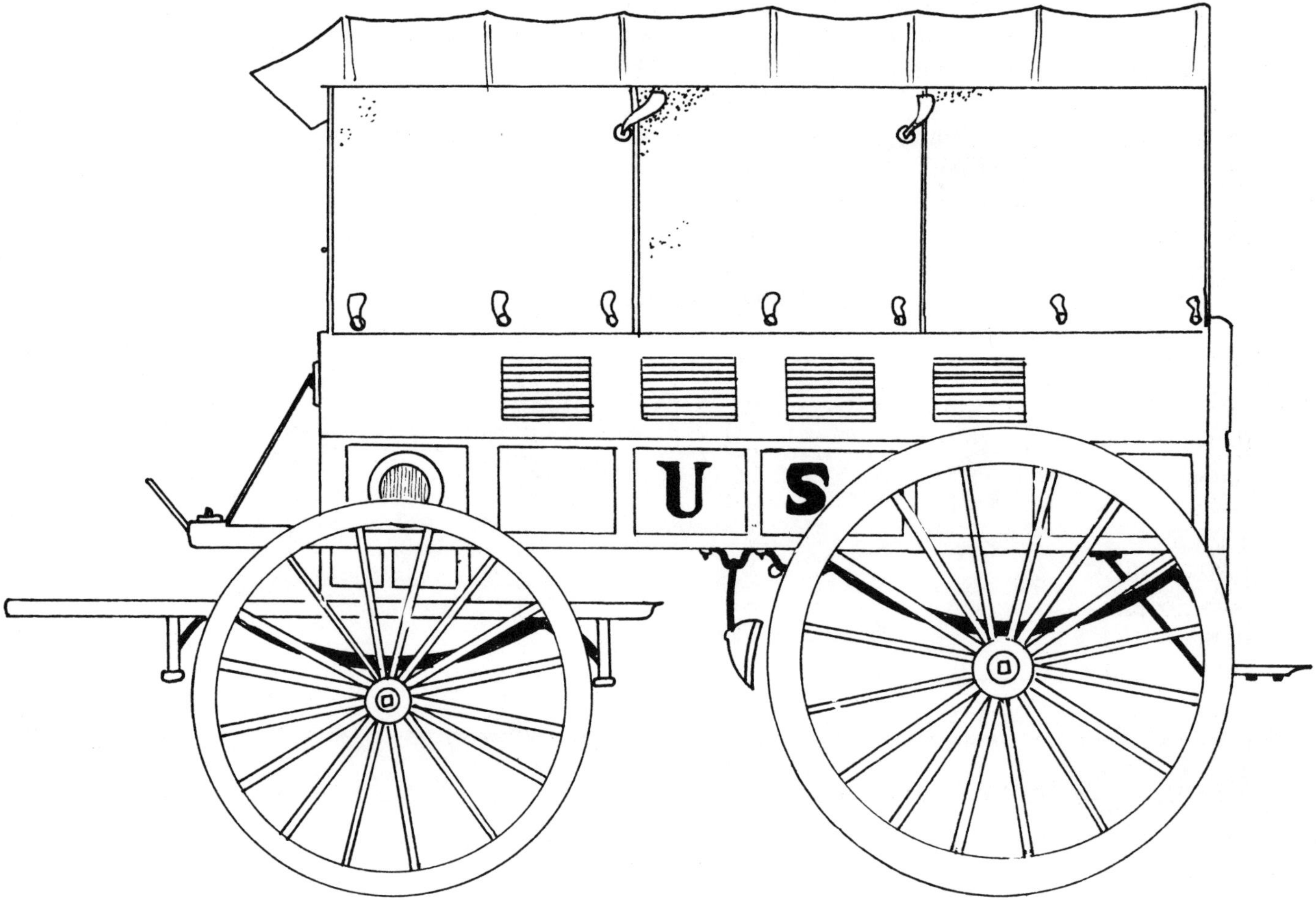

Figure 5-18, The Rucker Ambulance Wagon (side view)

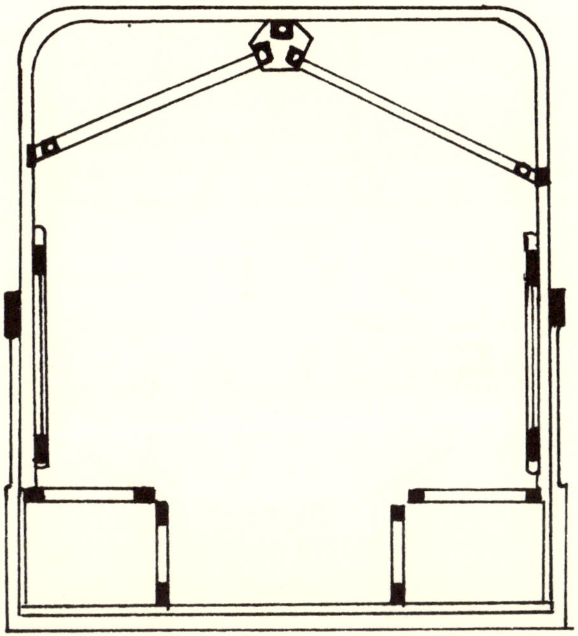

Figure 5-18a, The Rucker for ordinary use

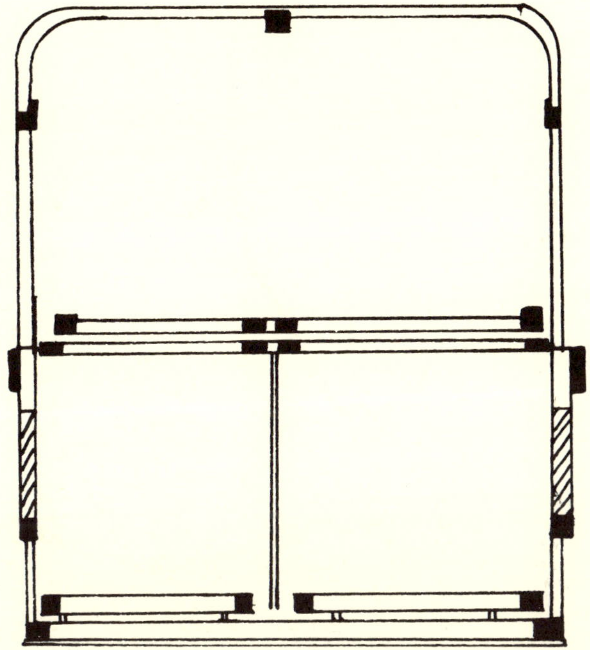

Figure 5-18b, The Rucker for patients, recumbent

Figures 5-17 through 5-20

Redrawn from *Medical-Surgical History, War of Rebellion,* Part III, Vol. II

Because of its weight and the four horses needed to pull it, efforts were made to design a lighter, more maneuverable wagon which could carry a fair number of wounded. The WHEELING, or ROSECRANS, was the result. This ambulance was, at first, built in the government shops at Wheeling, West Virginia (hence its name), after a design of General W.S. Rosecrans. This ambulance was much lighter than the Tripler and could accommodate twelve men sitting or two lying down, and three or four sitting.

The Wheeling (Figure 5-16)

Sills - 8'6" long, out to out (incuding foot board; 2 1/2" wide x 1 3/4" deep. Best quality ash.

Body- 7'6" long, 4' wide. Bottom 1/2" pine boards. Depth 23 1/2"; headroom 4'6"; board on front bow 12" wide; door back of body 21" wide. Framework of best quality white oak, thoroughly seasoned. The bows for top covering of ash. Cover of ambulance, front and back curtain, No. 4 duck; 3 roll-up curtains each side of body.

From the records examined, it appeared that the Philadelphia firms took most of the ambulance manufacturing business, followed by Cincinnati and New York City. Some of the Philadelphia firms were Henry Simon, Jacob Rech, Wilson Childs & Co., W.H. Ernst, Kneass & Co., N.L. Hart, J.B. Eldridge and M.W. Woods. Cincinnati was represented by such firms as Willis Baden, Phillip Dom, S. Peacock & Co., H. Ohlsen, F. Boise and Benjamin R. Stevens.

We have been describing the four-wheeled ambulance wagons that saw action during the Civil War. It is time to take a glimpse at a few patterns that didn't make it. Some of these had peculiar features that rendered them interesting, but not enough to make them effective. One was a four-wheeled ambulance designed by Assistant Surgeon

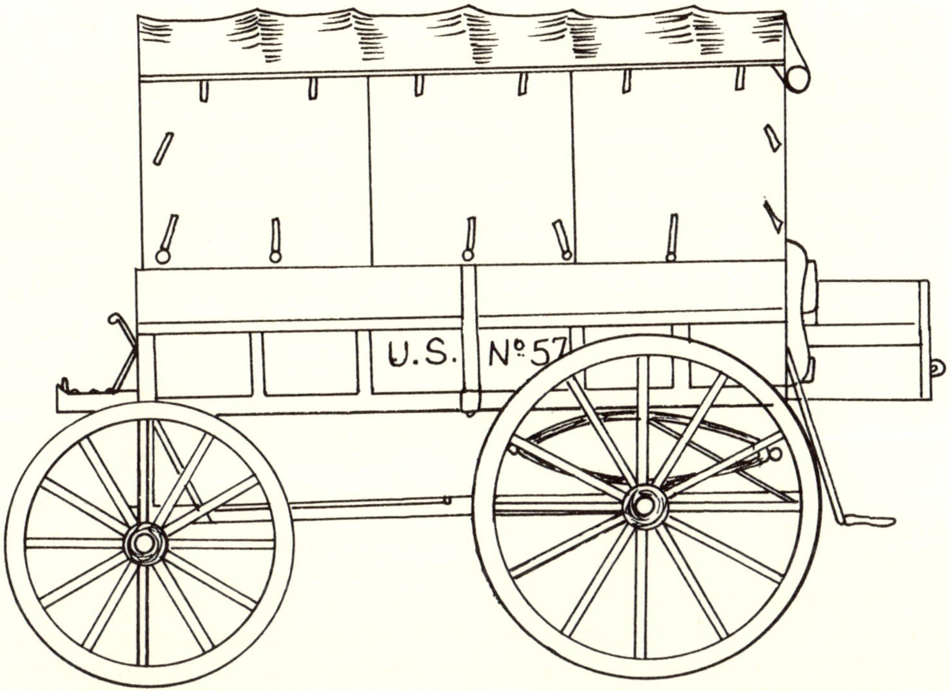

Figure 5-16, The Wheeling or Rosecrans Ambulance Wagon (side view)

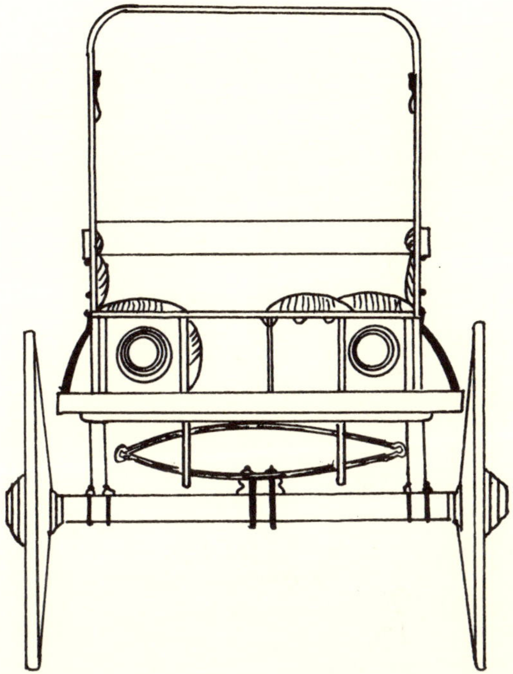

Figure 5-16a, The Wheeling (rear view)

Redrawn from *Medical-Surgical History, War of Rebellion,* Part III, Vol. II

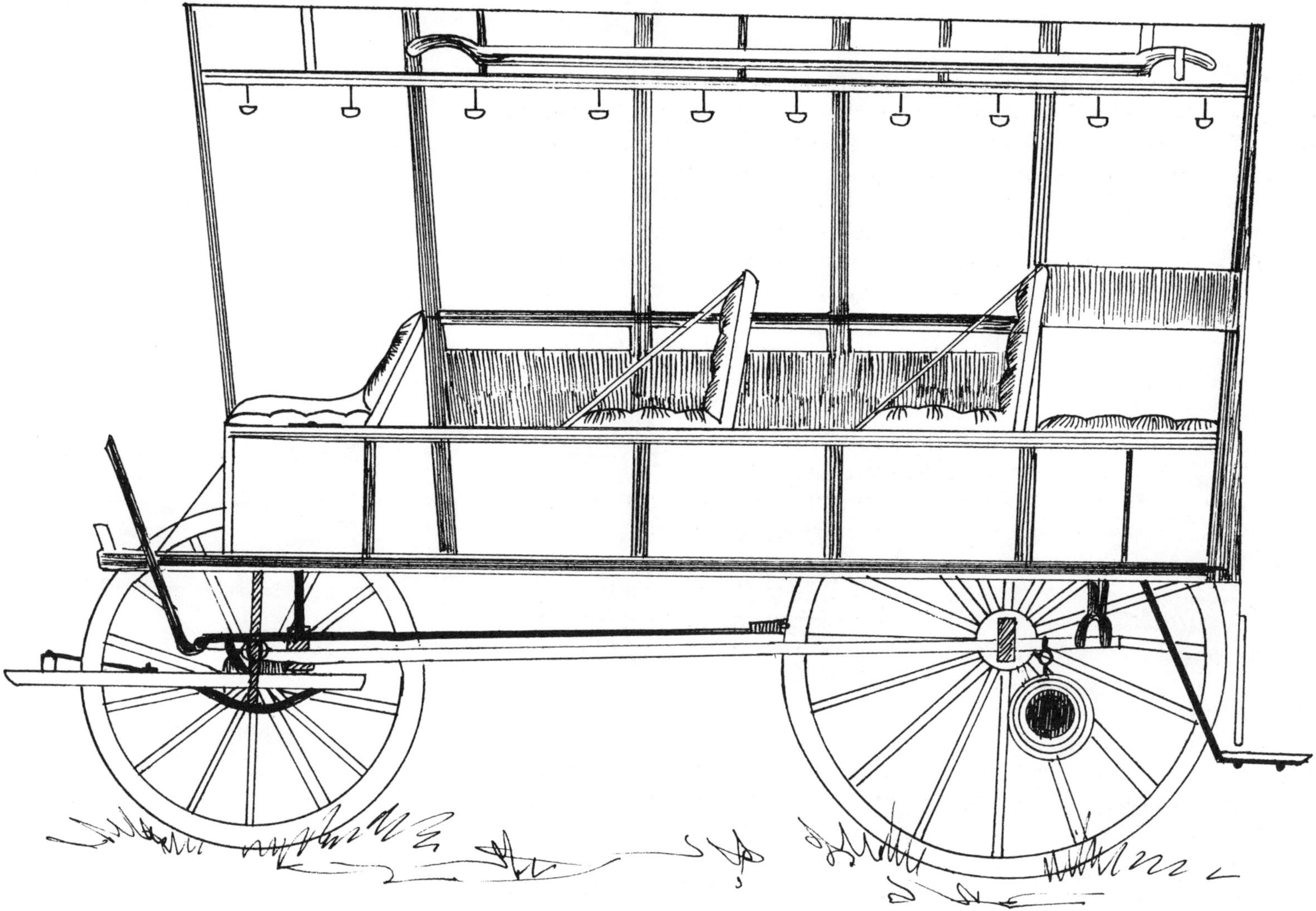

Figure 5-17, New Coolidge Ambulance Wagon arranged for sitting patients (cut away side view)
Redrawn from *Medical-Surgical History, War of Rebellion,* Part III, Vol. II

R.H. Coolidge who had designed one of the two-wheelers used during the early 1860s. This Coolidge four-wheeler was large, and therefore, heavy. The sills measured 10'4" in length; the body rested on 7"-9-¾" elliptical springs, placed on the outside of the wagon frame which was supposed to make it ride easier. It was intended to accommodate ten patients. This rather cumbersome vehicle was little used.[15]

In October, 1864, Assistant Surgeon Howard constructed an ambulance wagon for which he claimed many advantages such as:

1. Two wooden litters for seriously wounded.
2. Six permanent seats—corner seats provided with backs and cushions which tended to prevent the patients from being jostled about.
3. To minimize rolling, pitching and jolting, the body of the ambulance rested on semi-elliptical springs.
4. The platform for the litters rested on springs which tended to take up some of the shock from ordinary jolting.
5. Water tanks replaced kegs.
6. A large number of medical supplies could be stored in the vehicle without interfering with the comfort of the patients.

The weight of the ambulance was 1,232 pounds empty, a bit more than ambulances then in use. Nevertheless, the Board recommended that each army division be furnished two of the Howards and that a number of the older ambulances be altered to comply with the Howard. But, after nine months experience in the field, this ambulance failed to live up to expectations. It was heavy and cumbersome; it required four horses to draw it; and it was so complicated that it always got out of commission.

Toward the end of 1864, Dr. Langer proposed an ambulance wagon with so many radical changes and ingenious devices that the

Board of Officers turned it down as too complicated to withstand the test of field service.[16]

Like the proverbial plague of locusts, the ambulance inventors continued to besiege the offices of the War Department with their creations.

One such was a Mr. A.W. Siis (June, 1863), who asked the Board of Ambulance Examiners to see his product. They saw it, they disapproved. Mr. Siis, not to be so easily put off, came back a year later—same results, no approval. That took care of him, but soon after, Mr. G.W. Arnold appeared on the scene with his model. His idea was to use wooden litters. They were too heavy for practical use. No approval for him.

In the fall of 1864, Mr. E.R. McKean could have been seen coming down the pike with his "ideal" ambulance wagon. In his wagon, the litters were to be suspended from rubber rings. In addition, McKean's ambulance had contrivances fastened to the wheels so that the turning of the wheels forced air up into the interior of the ambulance. The Board thought the litter suspension idea a good one, but the ambulance had too many mechanical features which could get out of order, hence, no approval.

Even women got into the act. Whether or not she ever approached the War Department with her ambulance design, Claressa Britain of St. Joseph, Michigan, obtained a patent on her uniquely designed ambulance wagon.

In September 1865, the Medical Board of Officers was convened again to examine an Indian rubber spring ambulance wagon brought to its attention by Perot & Company of Philadelphia. The Board was very favorably impressed with this wagon. They thought that the India rubber springs were superior to the steel springs. An ambulance built upon this plan, belonging to the West Philadelphia Fire Company, was

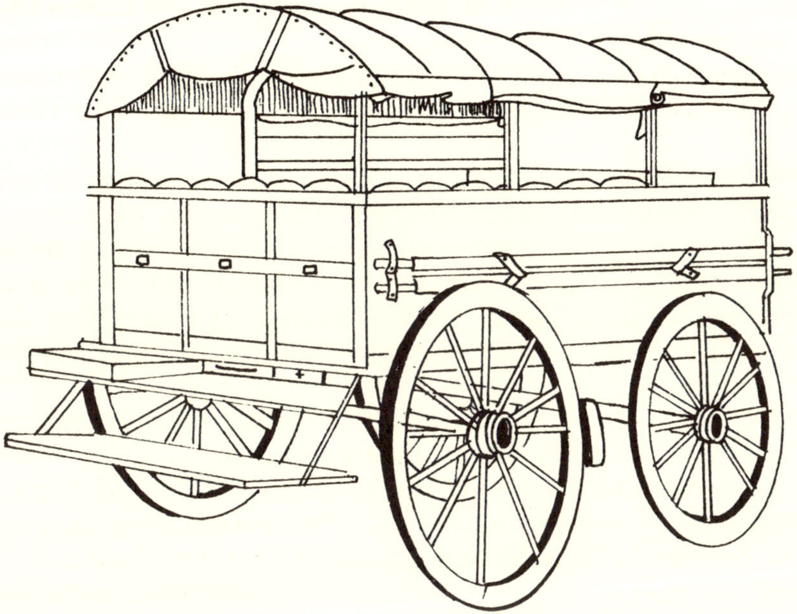

Figure 5-19, The Howard Ambulance Wagon

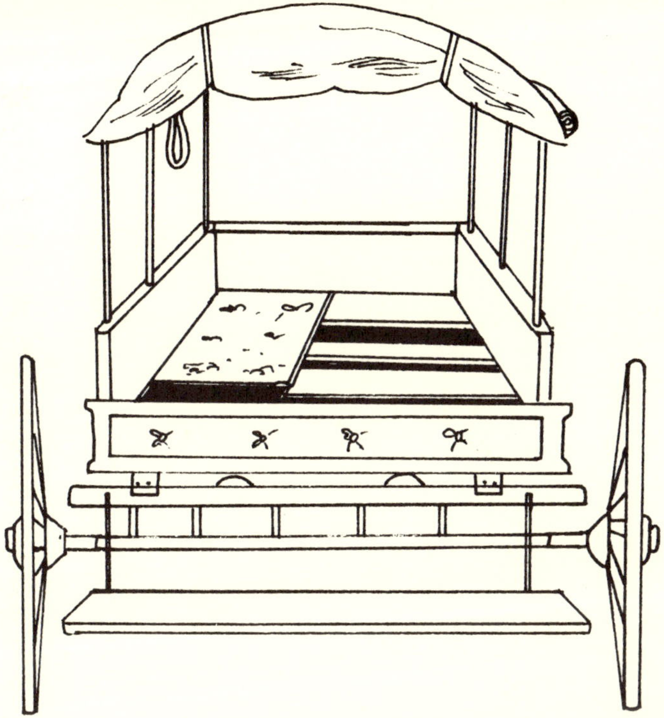

Figure 5-19a, The Howard (rear view)

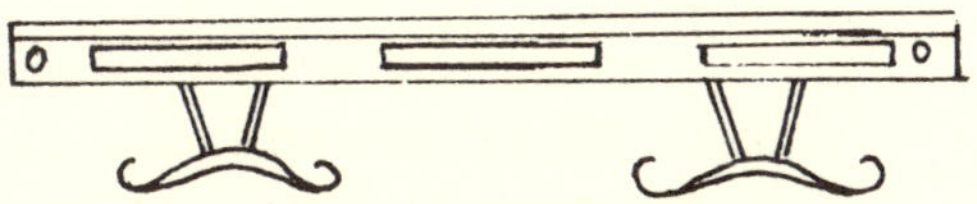

Figure 5-19b, Spring for bed or litter frame

shown to the Board. This ambulance had been in use for five years and showed little evidence of wear on the India rubber springs. India rubber springs could be replaced more easily and more quickly than the conventional steel springs. They weighed less, too, only 35¾ pounds, compared to the steel springs' 200 pounds for the same power. Cost, too, was much less, 27 dollars as opposed to 40 dollars. Records do not show that this model was ever adopted.[17]

As this chapter is brought to a close, the most important step forward in the transportation of the wounded troops was taken during the Civil War. Great improvements in design and construction were made. The Ruckers and the Wheelings were sound, serviceable vehicles which followed the armies westward to take their rightful place among the old standbys—the travois and the two-horse litters.

These tried and true vehicles gave way to the "Red Cross" pattern of 1878 which, in turn, was replaced, during World War I, by motorized ambulances, until today, we have the true "Flying Ambulances" in the shape of the Air Evac helicopters.

So it is now time to close the book on the litters, cacolets, ambulance wagons and the men who gave them substance with the sincere hope that through these pages some of their story will be remembered.

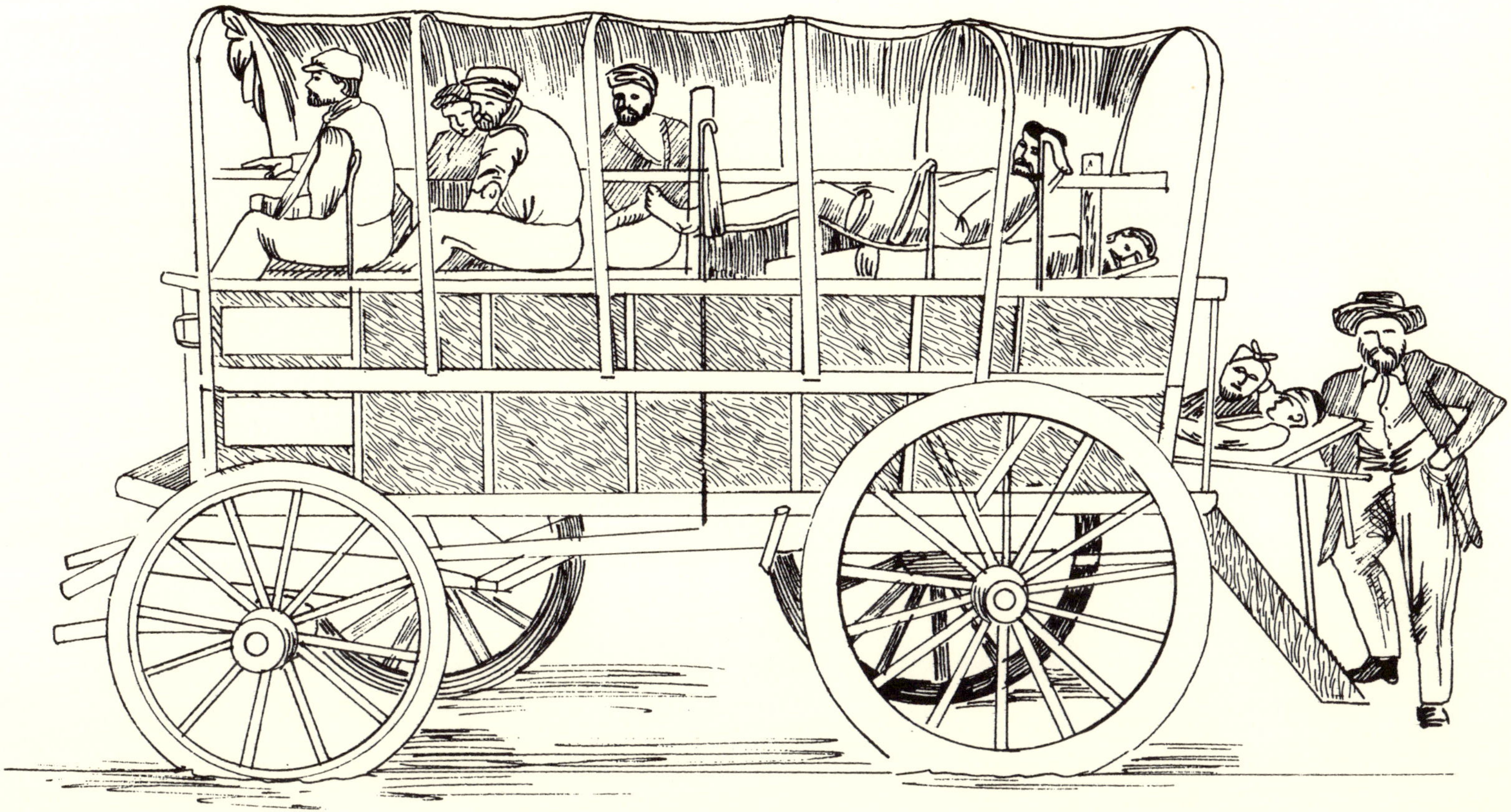

Figure 5-20, Army Wagon fitted up as an ambulance

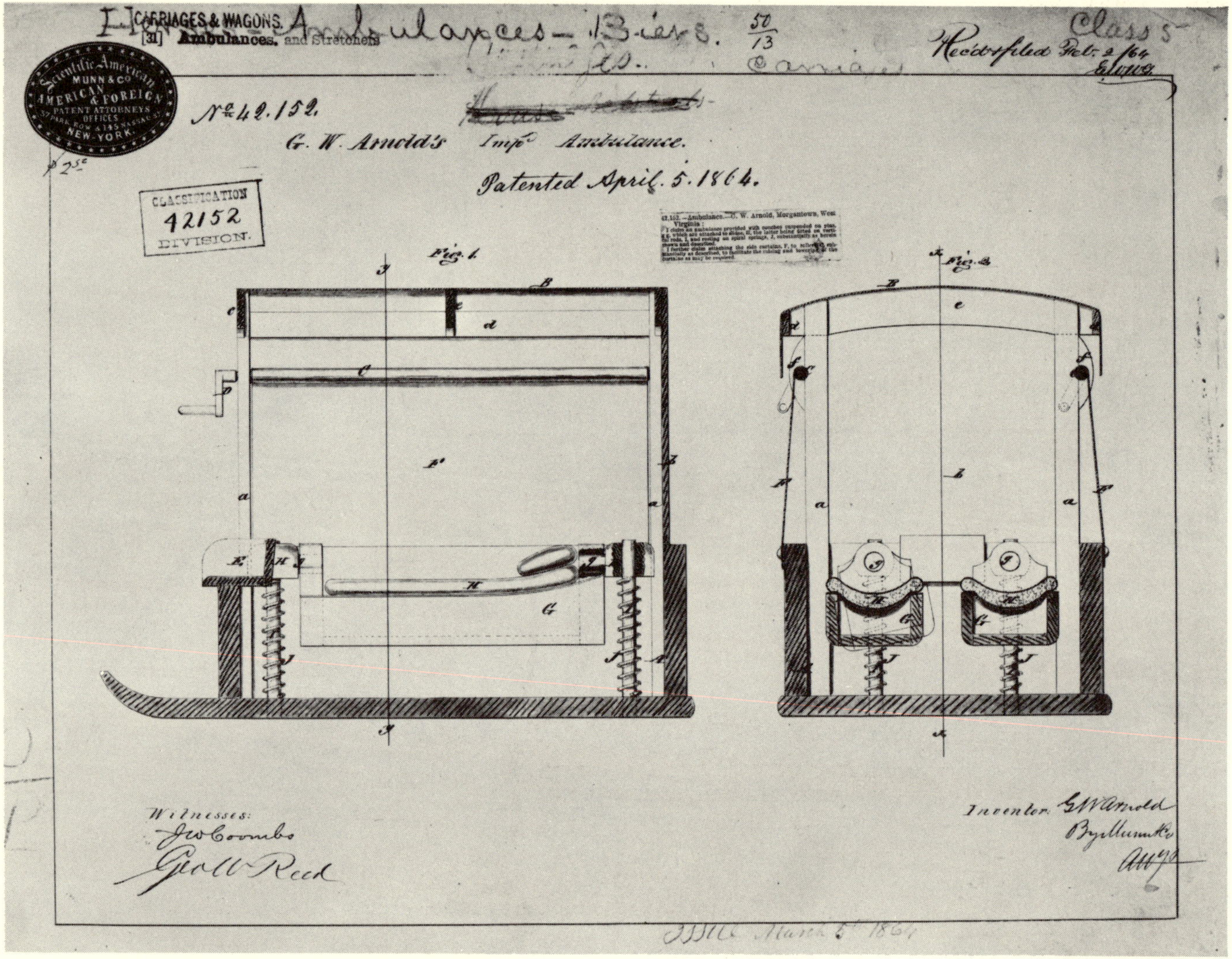

Figure 5-21, Patent drawing of G.W. Arnold's "Improved" Ambulance, *courtesy, National Archives*

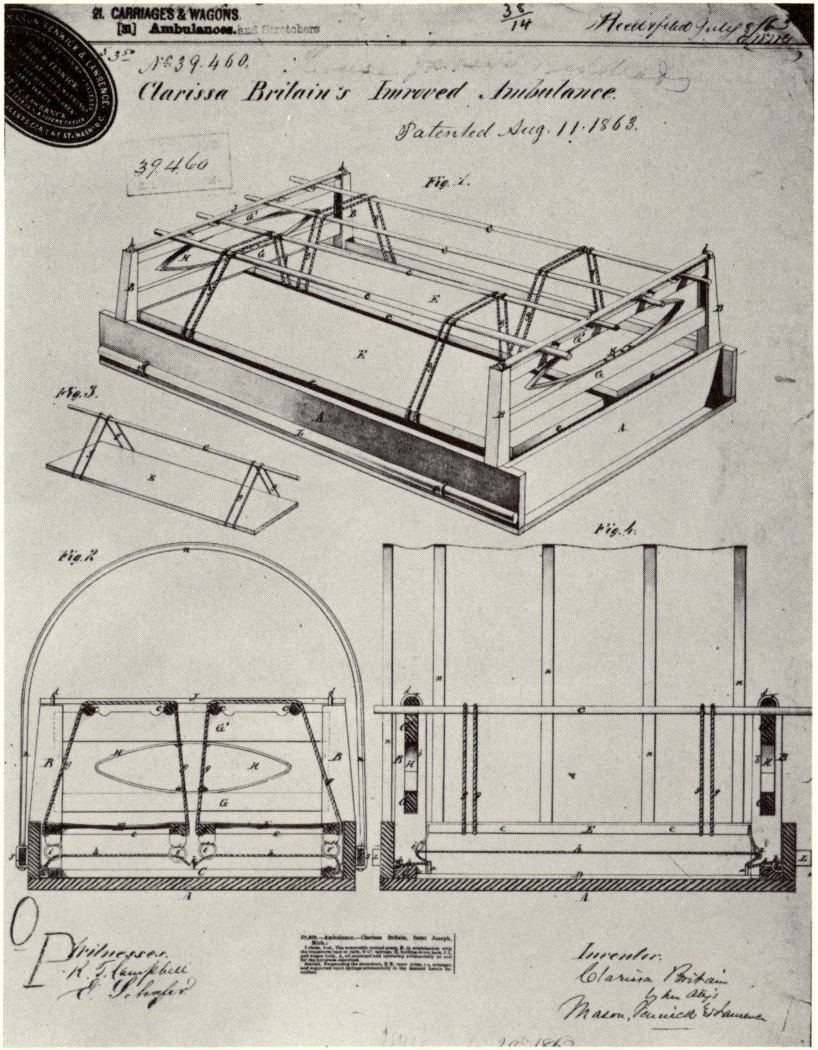

Figure 5-23, Patent drawing of Claressa Britain's "Improved" Ambulance
courtesy, National Archives

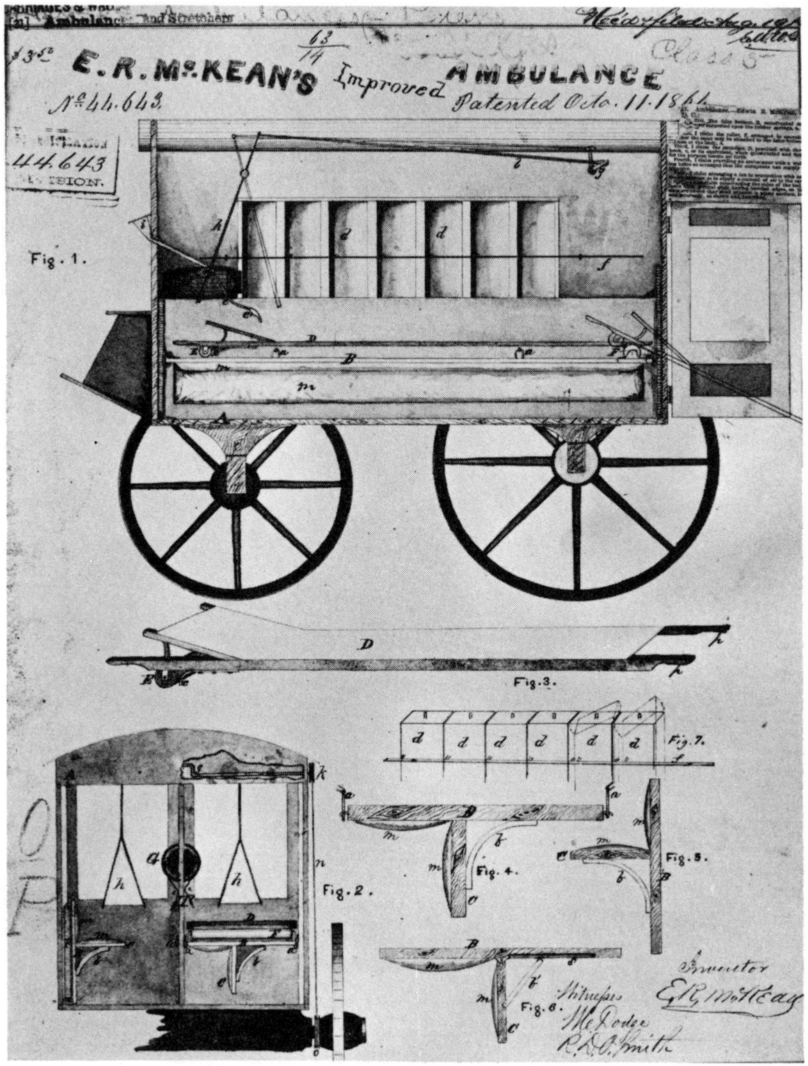

Figure 5-22, Patent drawing of E.R. McKean's "Improved" Ambulance *courtesy, National Archives*

Chapter V
NOTES

Section One

1. Gordon, Charles A., *Army Hygiene*, John Churchill and Sons, London (1863), p. 230.
2. War Department, The Surgeon General's Office, *The Medical and Surgical History of the War of the Rebellion*, Part III, Vol. II, p. 923 (hereinafter referred to as OR.).
3. OR., p. 924.
4. OR., p. 924.
5. OR., p. 925.

Section Two

1. OR., p. 926.
2. Longmore, Sir Thomas, *Treatise on Transport of Sick and Wounded Troops*, His Majesty's Stationery Office, London (1866), p. 213.

Section Three

1. War Department, Army Regulations, 1861 Revised par. 1298.
2. Longmore, *Treatise*, p. 293.
3. Marcy, General Randolph B., *The Prairie Traveler*, p. 150.
4. Otis, p. 6.
5. Ibid., p. 26.
6. Ibid., p. 5.
7. *Office of the Quartermaster General*, Letters Sent, Quartermaster General Thomas Jesup (Nov. 9, 1839), Record Group 92, Entry 289 (National Archives and Research Service).
8. Longmore, *Treatise*, p. 272.
9. Otis, General George A., "Transportation of Sick and Wounded by

Pack Animal," *War Department, The Surgeon General's Office,* Circular No. 9 (1877), p. 7.

10. Otis, pp. 8, 9.
11. Hamilton, Frank H., *A Treatise on Military Surgery and Hygiene,* Bailliere Bros., New York City (1865), p. 162.
12. Otis, p. 10.
13. Otis, p. 28.
14. Otis, pp. 15, 16.

Section Four

1. OR., pp. 944-946.
2. *Office of the Quartermaster General,* "Consolidated Correspondence File, 1794-1915," RG 92, Entry 1262, Box 30 (National Archives and Record Service).
3. *Office of the Quartermaster General,* "Register of Contracts," RG 92, Entry 1238, Volume 14 (NARS).
4. RG. 92, Entry 1262, Box 30.
5. RG. 92, Entry 1262, Box 30.
6. RG. 92, Entry 1262, Box 30.
7. RG. 92, Entry 1262, Box 30.
8. RG. 92, Entry 1238, Vol. 14.
9. RG. 92, Entry 1262, Box 31.
10. United States Secretary of War, *Annual Report 1865,* House Ex Document, 38th Congress 2d. Session.
11. RG. 92, Entry 1238, Vol. Year 1864.
12. RG. 92, Entry 1262, Box 31.
13. RG. 92, Entry 1262, Box 30.
14. RG. 92, Entry 1238, Vols. 14, 15.
15. *Medical and Surgical History of the War of the Rebellion,* Part III, Vol. II, p. 950.
16. *Medical and Surgical History,* pp. 954, 955.
17. *Medical and Surgical History,* p. 952.

Appendix

MEDICINE WAGONS

One of the most important links in the chain of supply from Medical Purveyors to the surgeons in the field and to the medicine boxes under the ambulance driver's seat was the medicine wagon.

At the beginning of the war, each regimental surgeon was furnished with suitable equipment for his regiment for field service, consisting of medicine, stores, instruments and dressings in quantities regulated by the Standard Supply Table. In action, he was accompanied by a hospital orderly who carried a knapsack containing a limited supply of anaesthetics, styptics, stimulants and anodynes, and material for primary dressings. The knapsack wasn't really a sack; it was a wicker-work style box covered with enamelled cloth (Figure 6-3), 18 inches high, 15 inches wide, by 7½ inches deep; weight when filled was 18 pounds. The contents of the knapsack might be of interest. They were: 1 piece of white wax, 8 oz. simple cerate, 12 oz. chloroform, 5 yds. adhesive plaster, 2 yds. isinglass plaster, 1 oz. persulfate of iron, 100 compound cathartic pills, 150 blue mass pills, 150 opium and camphor pills, 150 quinine pills, 8 oz. aromatic spirits of ammonia, 16 oz. brandy, 4 oz. laudenum, 10 bandages, 14 binder boards, 4 oz. charpie, 2 medium glasses, 1 (spirit) lamp, 12 oz. lint, 1 box matches, 1 paper of pins, 1 spool surgical silk, 4 pieces sponge, 4 (Dunton's) field tourniquets, 2 spinal tourniquets, 1 piece tape, 1 spool of lead wire, 1 spool of silver wire, and 1 spatula.

The hospital medicine chest, mess chest and bulky hospital supplies were transported in heavy supply wagons which were, all too often, not readily accessible when required. To overcome this serious problem, panniers were provided containing the necessary medicines, dressings and appliances. These panniers were designed to be carried on the backs of animals, but were found to be too heavy and thus were more generally carried in one of the ambulances. Figures 6-4 and 6-4a show a pannier designed by Dr. Squibb of Brooklyn, New York. It consisted of a strong box 21-1/8" long, 11-3/4" wide and 11-3/8" deep. When filled, it weighed a considerable 88 pounds.

To overcome this weight problem and to have medical supplies at hand, Surgeon Jonathan Letterman, who succeeded Surgeon Tripler as Medical Director of the Army of the Potomac, induced the firm of E. Hayes and Company of Wheeling, West Virginia, to construct a medicine wagon of his design. It had been unanimously approved by a medical board of officers, but unfortunately, details of this particular wagon could not be obtained.

In the late fall of 1862, Mr. J. Dunton proposed a medicine wagon, but it was turned down by a board of examiners as being poorly constructed and too small to carry a three months supply of regimental hospital stores.

But, as the war progressed, the medical organization was, providentially, reorganized along brigade lines rather than regimental, and each brigade was provided with a medicine wagon which carried, in addition to an ample supply of drugs, dressings, medical furniture and appliances, as well as an amputating table. The contents of the medicine wagons were constantly replenished from the Brigade Medical Purveyor's stores.

It wasn't until rather late in the war though (June, 1864), that the Medical Department received the Autentrieth medicine wagon (Figure 6-2). Nine such wagons were initially built at the Schuykill Arsenal. This wagon held one distinct advantage over the earlier models—medical stores did not have to be packed, and then unpacked. It saved much hauling and pulling of medicine boxes.

(Material for this appendix taken from "Medical and Surgical History of the War of the Rebellion," Part III, Vol. II, pp. 914-918.)

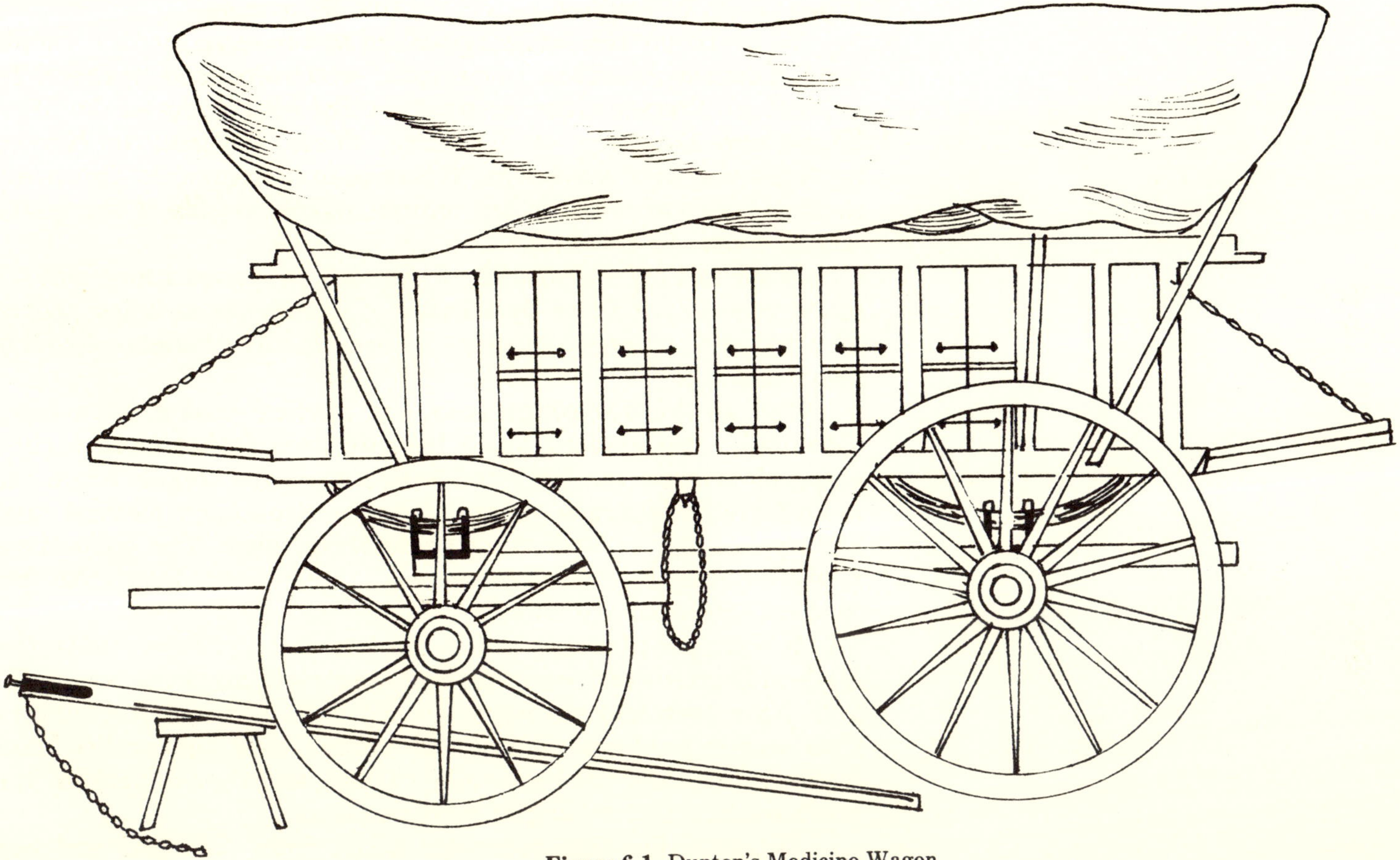

Figure 6-1, Dunton's Medicine Wagon

Figures 6-1 through 6-4a
Redrawn from *Medical-Surgical History, War of Rebellion,* Part III, Vol. II

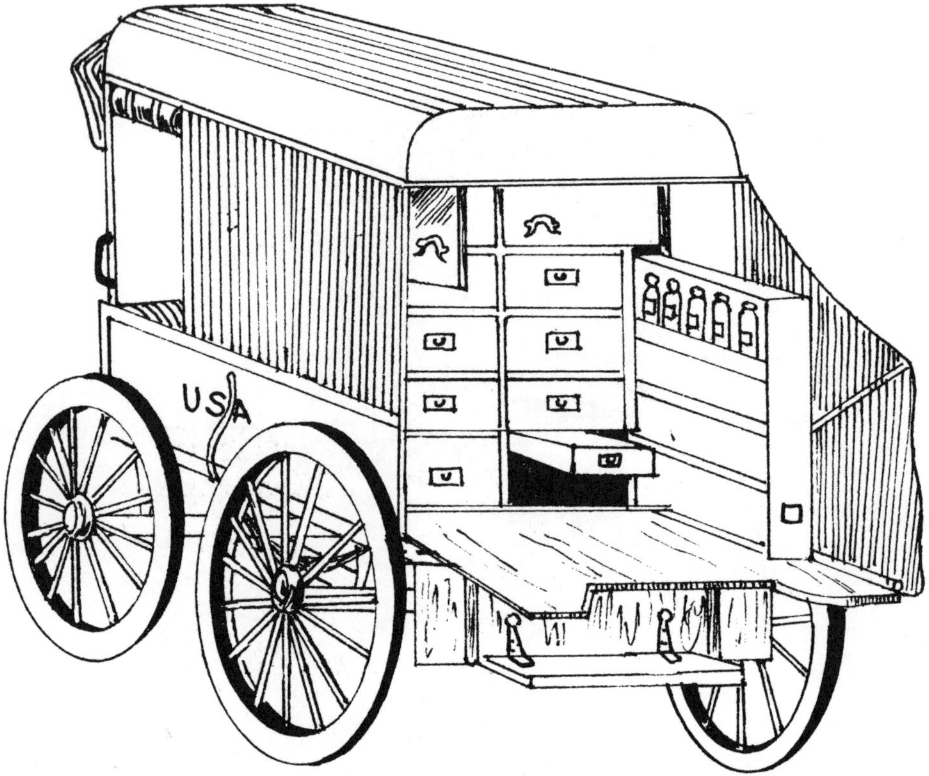

Figure 6-2, Autentrieth Medicine Wagon

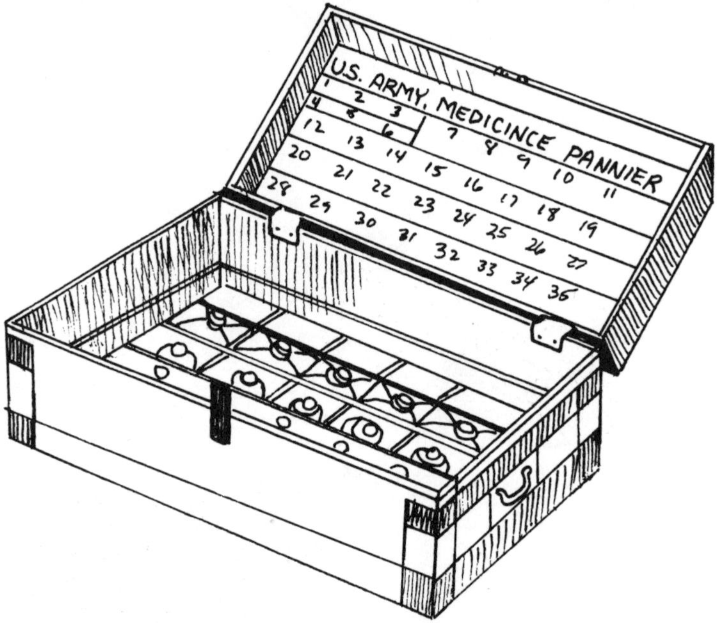

Figure 6-4, Medicine Pannier

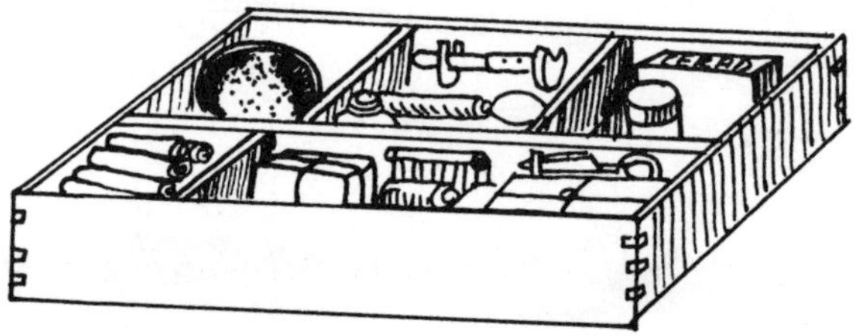

Figure 6-4a, Upper Tray Medicine Pannier

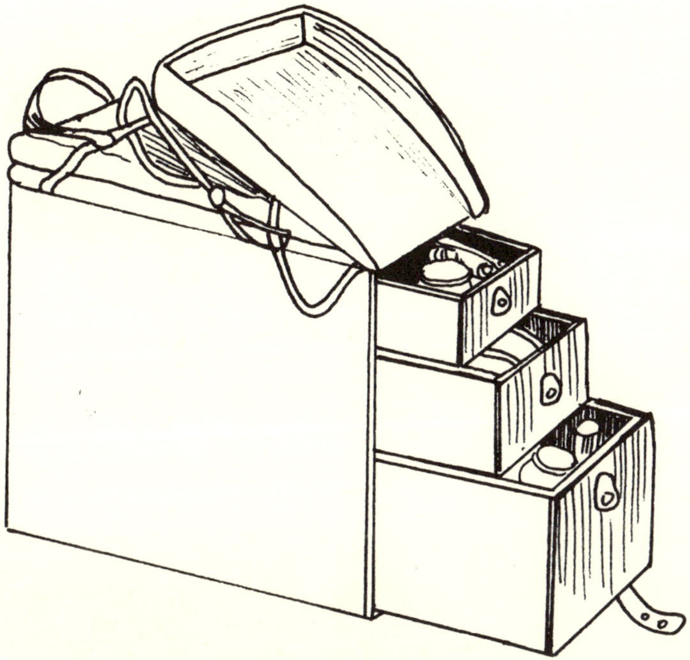

Figure 6-3, Hospital Knapsack (wicker work)

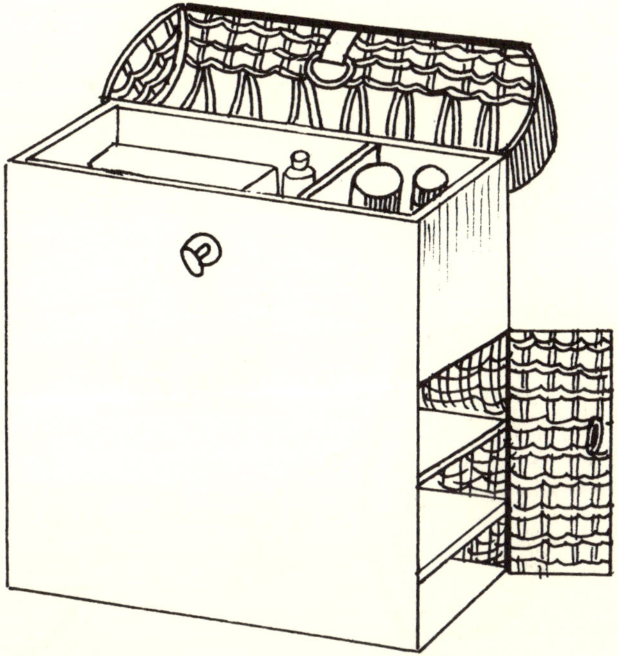

Figure 6-3a, Regulation Hospital Knapsack, 1862

BIBLIOGRAPHY

GENERAL BIBLIOGRAPHY

Published Documents

Brown, Harvey E., *The Medical Department of the United States Army, 1775-1873*, Washington, Government Printing Office, 1873.

Heitman, Frances B., *Historical Register and Dictionary of the United States Army, 1789-1903*, Vol. I, Washington, Government Printing Office, 1903.

Hershler, Nathaniel, *The Soldier's Handbook*, Washington, Government Printing Office, 1884.

Otis, General George A., *Transporting of Sick and Wounded by Pack Animals*, War Department, The Surgeon General's Office Circular No. 9, Washington, Government Printing Office, 1877.

Upton, General Emory, *The Military Policy of the United States*, Washington, Government Printing Office, 1907.

War Department, *Revised Army Regulations, 1861*, Washington, Government Printing Office, 1861.

War Department, The Surgeon General's Office, *The Medical and Surgical History of the War of the Rebellion, 1861-65*, Part III, Vol. II, Washington, 1883.

United States Secretary of War, *Annual Report, 1865*, House Executive Document, 38th Congress, 2d. Session.

United States Congress, Senate Executive Document No. 59, 36th Congress, 1st Session, 1860, "Report On The Art of War in Europe, 1854-56," by Major Richard Delafield.

Unpublished Documents

Adjutant General's Office, *Consolidated Correspondence File, Letters Received*, "General Terry to Assistant Adjutant Division of the Missouri, December 7, 1876," RG 94, Entry 622, Washington,

National Archives and Research Service.
Office of the Quartermaster General, *Consolidated Correspondence File, 1794-1915*, RG 92, Entry 1262, Boxes 30, 31, Washington, National Archives and Research Service.
Office of the Quartermaster General, *Letters Sent*, QMG. Thomas Jesup, 1839-1840, RG. 92, Entry 289, National Archives and Research Service.
Office of the Quartermaster General, "Register of Contracts," RG. 92, Entry 1328, Vol. 14-16, Washington, National Archives and Research Service.

Secondary Sources

Adams, George W., *Doctors In Blue*. New York City, Macmillan and Co., 1952.
Ashburn, Percy M., *A History of the Medical Department of the U.S. Army*. New York City, Houghton-Mifflin Company, 1929.
Brooks, Stewart, *Civil War Medicine*. Springfield, Illinois, Charles C. Thomas, 1966.
Callan, John F., *Military Laws of the United States, 1777-1863*, 2d. Edition, Philadelphia, George W. Childs, 1863.
Cunningham, Horace H., *Doctors In Gray*. Baton Rouge, La., Louisiana State University, 1958.
Dictionary of American Bibliography. Allen Johnson and Dumas Malone, Editors, Vols. IV, IX. New York City, Charles Scribner's and Sons, 1930.
Drum, William F., "Work of the Fifth Ambulance Train" in *Glimpses of the Nation's Struggles*, 3d. Series, Edward Neill, Editor. New York City, D.D. Merrill and Company, 1893.
Duncan, Lt. Col. Louis C., *The Medical Department of the U.S. Army*

In The Civil War, no publisher, 1914. (A series of articles written for and used by the Medical Department, U.S. Army.)

Duncan, Lt. Col. Louis C., *Medical Men In The Revolution, 1775-1783*, Army Medical Bulletin No. 25, Medical Field Service Schools, Carlisle Barracks, Penn., 1931.

Gordon, Charles A., *Army Hygiene*, London, John Churchill and Sons, 1866.

Grace, William, *The Army Surgeon's Manual.* New York City, Bailliere Bros., 1864. (Published by permission of the Surgeon General.)

Graham, Colonel W.A., *The Custer Myth.* New York City, Bonanza Books, 1953.

Hamilton, Frank H., *A Treatise On Military Surgery and Hygiene.* New York City, Bailliere Bros., 1865.

Kimball, Maria B., *A Soldier Doctor of Our Army.* Boston, Houghton-Mifflin, 1917.

Letterman, Major Jonathan B., *Medical Recollections of the Potomac.* New York City, D. Appleton, 1866. (Microfilm Reel 169.6, University of Michigan, Ann Arbor.)

Longmore, General Sir Thomas, *A Treatise on the Transportation of Sick and Wounded Troops.* London, Her Majesty's Stationery Office, 1866. (Microfilm, History of Medicine, Division of National Library, Bethesda, Md.)

Marcy, General Randolph B., *The Prairie Traveler; A Handbook for Overland Expeditions, 1859.* New York City, Harper Bros., 1859.

Richardson, Robert G., *Larrey, Surgeon to Napoleon's Imperial Guard.* London, John Murray, 1974.

Rickey, Don., Jr., *Forty Miles A Day On Beans and Hay.* Norman, Oklahoma, University of Oklahoma Press, 1963.

Tobey, James A., *The Medical Department of the Army.* Baltimore, Md., John Hopkins Press, 1927. (Institute for Government Research Monograph No. 5.)

THE OLD ARMY PRESS